Stopping Abortions

at Death's Door

"In this book, Rod Murphy presents his plan to have a pregnancy resource center, with volunteers trained in sidewalk counseling, in close proximity to every abortion facility in the country. Rod calls on his wealth of experience on the front lines of this battle to explain just why the pro-life movement must implement this strategy and then gives details on all the aspects of starting this ministry in your town. I wholeheartedly agree with Rod on the efficacy of this approach and encourage everyone to read this book."
Jim Sedlak, *founder of STOPP International (Stop Planned Parenthood) & VP of American Life League, Stafford, VA*

"Roderick Murphy's new book is just what the pro-life movement needs: a clear, practical and realistic guide to the *direct* saving of human lives—at the doors of abortion clinics. After over 30 years running a non-profit pregnancy center in Worcester, Massachusetts, Murphy has extensive knowledge of how pregnancy centers and sidewalk counseling can be effective; with this new, invaluable resource, he invites all pro-life Americans to help realize his dream to "put pregnancy centers next door to abortionists all over America."
Maria McFadden Editor, *Human Life Review New York, NY*

Rod Murphy has focused decades of experience in every area of the pro-life movement to create and maintain the most successful crisis pregnancy center in New England. Written in sensible, comprehensible fashion, <u>Stopping Abortion at Death's Door</u> provides practical, proven methods for the most effective ways to save the lives of individual babies and to rescue their mothers from lives of heartbreak."
Anne Fox, President, *Massachusetts Citizens for Life,* Director, *National Right to Life Committee*

"Revolutionary . . . a must-have book for pregnancy care centers. Sound Wave Images did an ultrasound training at Problem Pregnancy in 2000 - great nurses and counselors. Rod speaks from the heart and has years of experience working with centers. He is also very entertaining and compelling. One minute he'll have you laughing and the next you are on the verge of tears. Great guy and Rod knows what he's writing about."
Shari Richard, *Sound Wave Images, West Bloomfield, MI*

Stopping Abortions at Death's Door

A Non-Violent System for Christians & Pro-Life Pregnancy Centers to Lawfully Battle for Babies' Lives at Abortion Facilities

Roderick P. Murphy

Taig Publishing

Southbridge, Massachusetts 01550

Also by Roderick P. Murphy

Growing Up, Unwashed

Taig Publishing 2009

Guidebook to Buying and Using a Vapor Degreaser

Taig Publishing 2004

Dedicated to the thousands of Massachusetts mothers who choose life over abortion for their babies. And all the wonderful Problem Pregnancy woman counselors, inside and outside throughout our 28 year history, especially to Kathy Lake, the champion baby saver.

In Memoriam

I ask for God's mercy on all former Problem Pregnancy board members, counselors and volunteers, now deceased. They were pro-life pioneers.

Mary Mulcahy

James Walsh M.D.

John Spillane Esq.

Louise Auger

Frank Macey

Mary Russell

Helen Flaherty

Al Thoman

Mary Ram

Peggy O'Shea

Paul O'Leary M.D.

Msgr. Leo Battista

Ann Marie Blute

Patricia Taylor

I ask God's mercy on these three people who helped me form my strong antipathy towards abortion:

- *Sr. Marie St. James, my eighth grade teacher who explained to her 12 year old boys what a horror abortion is.*

- *Helen and Thomas Murphy, my wonderful parents who realized that abortion is a violent and deadly assault on innocent unborn babies and passed that realization on to me.*

Acknowledgments

Many people deserve acknowledgment and thanks for their help with this book. A writer needs people telling him what's right and especially what's wrong with his manuscript. My critics were Ellen Murphy, Jean Murphy, Jennifer Murphy, Ursula Murphy, Charlie Coudert and Anne Fox. Some folks who helped with research or allowed their work to be used within the book are; Rita Nealon, Rose Thoman, Anne Scheidler, Jim Sedlak, Monsignor Philip Reilly and Professor Jon Shields and Professor Hadley Arkes.

Since most of my CPC experience and knowledge comes from my years at Problem Pregnancy of Worcester, Inc., many thanks are owed to the 1982 founders and others. Mentioned are just a few: Gerry Russell, the first director, who paved the way; Peggy O'Shea and Laurie Letourneau, two dynamos; Rose Thoman and Rita Nealon, who ran our baby boutique every Wednesday for over 25 years; Fr. Dan Becker, our chaplain and Fr. Michael Roy, our good friend. Fr. Tony Kazarnowicz, our hero, stood in front of the Planned Parenthood abortion facility in Worcester for over twenty years with his processional crucifix staff. Many abortions were turned away by his simple and powerful witness. Captain Tony Kazarnowicz is now an Army chaplain and a veteran of the Iraq and Afghanistan Wars, another kind of hero.

Also without our generous donors, small and large, Problem Pregnancy would not exist. Thank you all!

Preface

Roderick P. Murphy, born in 1939, is a husband, father, grandfather, brother, uncle, and granduncle to a large Boston Irish family. He has spent over 50 years in American industry. He owns an industrial machinery sales firm and is a real estate developer in Southbridge, Massachusetts.

For over 40 years, starting even before the U.S. Supreme Court's Roe v. Wade decision, Rod has been fighting abortion. He has been instrumental in founding and running many pro-life, baby-saving organizations. For almost 30 years, he has been the leader of Problem Pregnancy, a non-profit pregnancy center in Worcester, Massachusetts. He is a strong believer in Jesus Christ Crucified, the Roman Catholic Church, family and America. He believes that God has smiled on him throughout his life.

Why Good People Should Read This Book

I am a 71-year-old American citizen, born in a three decker in Cambridge, Massachusetts. I am a husband, a father of six children and a grandfather of eight. I have five daughters and five sisters and work with mostly women. I am a businessman and a real estate developer. I served in the U.S. Army as a young man. I have never missed voting in an election and have been an elected delegate to two National

Republican Presidential Conventions. Like all of us, I am a sinner and I am a believing and active Roman Catholic.

On the other hand I have been told that I hate women, that I'm anti-choice and that I have a "fetus fetish". I've been called a religious zealot. I've been spat upon and assaulted on the public sidewalk. I've been jeered at, been flipped the bird and been battered by many passersby. I've been videotaped and harassed by police officers on city streets. I've been arrested on public ways and jailed. I've been listed on FBI watch lists as a potential domestic terrorist. I'm not allowed to walk on certain public sidewalks in Boston, Worcester, Brookline, Lynn, Springfield, Haverhill and Attleboro, Massachusetts and in many other cities and states. Protesting on the side of a state highway, I've had nasty liquids and solids thrown at me from passing cars. For 35 years my letters to the editor were spiked by biased newspaper editors. I've been stripped of my delegate credentials at a state Republican Convention by "pro-choicers"after being elected by voters. My state's newspapers, TV and radio stations and the other dominant media have not reported any of this unjust and unconstitutional treatment.

Why? Because I'm an implacable, unbending and long-term foe of the abortion of innocent human babies and the establishment and the media has been drafted by the opposing team. I'm aghast and indignant that millions of pre-born boys and girls are aborted every year in America. I'm aghast and indignant that all Americans are not equally aghast and indignant. I want Americans to get so angry at this massive slaughter of babies, that they storm the abortion mills like the angry Transylvanian mob in the movie at Dr. Frankenstein's gates, brandishing their torches, dogs and pitchforks. The difference would be that unlike the Transylvanians, we must be angry but peaceful. We must nonviolently stop this holocaust by putting our bodies and our intellect at the abortion front line.

I'm just one of hundreds of thousands of people who think that abortion is unconstitutional and ghastly to our little brothers and sisters who are treated with such merciless hate. I write about these insults, not for sympathy, but so readers will see, that I have credibility, what the young folks call "creds". I need you to pay attention for I have a national plan to stop abortions, right at death's door. I have written this book to explain my plan and to recruit other aghast and indignant Americans to help me implement it. Pick up your torches and pitchforks, leash up your pit-bulls and follow me through this book and then to the abortion mills.

1.

Wanted: Dedicated, selfless people with boundless energy, contagious personalities, and hearts of gold. Must be willing to save babies, help mothers and leap over buildings in a single bound. Most mere humans need not apply.

What's the Problem?

In the years since Roe v Wade, a slow incremental acceptance of abortion has occurred. In 1973 that Supreme Court decision was considered radical and not accepted by the majority of Americans. Today the attitude among aborting women has devolved down to—if it's legal, then it must be moral. This is an elementary philosophical error by a population, not given to deep thinking and while at the same time, looking for a quick solution to their own life-upsetting problem. That attitude, together with selfishness and pressure from boyfriends, parents and friends, causes pregnant women to abort their children over a million times each year in the U.S.A. Many women of childbearing age are promiscuously sleeping around, tempting pregnancy. When they almost inevitably get pregnant, this generation of women (and men) seems to think that killing this generation of babies by abortion is OK.

Those women, now pregnant, often have no support from families, boyfriends or friends. The individual woman gets no offsetting advice about the life and rights of the unborn baby. Many of her contacts pressure her to abort the child. The reasons given to abort are mostly trite but there are many of them. She is too young or she's still in school or the baby's father doesn't believe it's his or she has no way to raise a child or her apartment is too small or she will have to stop working toward the end of the pregnancy and can not afford that. The silent, defenseless baby can't compete with those excuses to destroy her.

At the same time, that these women are getting this barrage of one-sided, pro-abortion advice, we have a plague of voracious entrepreneurs in the abortion "business" all over the nation, trying to get these pregnant mothers into their "clinics" to chop up their babies at $650 apiece. They advertise in yellow pages, newspapers, on TV, on the internet, on buses and trains and in college newspapers. These sleazy abortionists have the morality of a cancer cell. The pregnant woman or her baby are of no concern, just the cash she brings to the abortion mill. Ms Magazine may find those bottom-feeders heroic but the truth is that abortionists are mendacious, mercenary and profoundly evil.

I view this abortion infestation with a lot of testosterone, as a man, as a husband, as a father and as a protector of my family. You might notice that I never use the word "pro-choice" in this book. I think that any policy having even the possibility of killing one little innocent human pre-born should be called pro-abortion not pro-choice. No option for abortion should be legal, according to the Declaration of Independence and the Fourteenth Amendment of the U.S. Constitution. You might also notice that I put quotation marks around the word "clinic" when it appears after the word abortion. A clinic is a place, where doctors try to heal and help people. Abortionists hurt and kill people.

Those mercenaries of death also have the great benefit of having many allies in the news media. I think there is a scandal within journalism regarding the obvious conflicts of interest among reporters on abortion. On many other stories, journalists might have no personal opinion one way or another but with abortion; many have a definite interest in keeping abortion legal and available. The median age of journalists is 41.

Many men use abortion to remain sexually active. The natural result of heterosexual promiscuity is pregnancy. Abortion is very convenient for men but traumatic for women. Legal abortion contributes to male irresponsibility with male journalists included. The minimalist morality today for a man is that he be a barely interested sperm donor and that when he impregnates, he pays for his female partner's aborting of his child. I include at least some reporters in this cohort of irresponsible, abortion-using men.

Of course women are reporters too and in today's world many of those women are having sex recreationally and sometimes they get pregnant. Male and female reporters seem to be comfortable knowing that abortion is available as a backup to contraception for their sexual activity. How can such writers be objective while covering abortion stories? The coverage is one-sided because the media functionaries are one sided. Editors must know about this obvious bias for abortion and the industry's ongoing conflict of interest.

Since 1973 almost never has the mainstream media treated the anti-abortion side fairly. Objectivity is a fancy word, used often in journalism classes but regarding abortion news, it never ventures beyond the classroom. The biggest offenders are the biggest news businesses; the New York Times, the Washington Post, the L.A. Times, the Chicago Tribune, the Boston Globe, ABC TV, CBS TV, NBC TV, AP, UPI, Reuters et al. No woman who watches TV or reads the newspaper would ever get a pro-life viewpoint, unless her TV breaks down and she goes next door to old Mrs. Kelly's to watch the weather and gets to see EWTN TV (a Catholic TV network) by mistake. Even the potentially diverse letters to the editor sections in newspapers too often spike pro-life letters; e.g. the Boston Globe never prints pro-life letters. The endangered baby never gets a break from the scribblers and the legions of TV blonds and pretty-boy TV newsreaders. Even the pro-aborts agree that they have the media in their Gucci handbags. Suzanne Millsaps of NARAL bragged as follows, "The media has been our best friend in this fight. They claim objectivity but I know they're all pro-choice".

All these unfortunate factors come together today when a woman has an unplanned pregnancy, a euphemism, if I ever heard one. How many pregnancies are really planned? Almost none. Those of us who find the destruction of humans to be abhorrent, are called pro-life. We pro-lifers have been fighting against all the above factors that make abortion appear to be the only choice to a pregnant woman. In spite of strong, pro-life efforts in many different ways, we are losing the battle for babies' lives 1.2 million* times a year and 52 million times since Roe v Wade. What do we do about it? I'll tell you but first let us look at the current pro-life offense and defense in this David vs. Goliath battle.

---

* Counting the number of abortions is complicated. The 1.2 million abortions per year and the 52 million abortions since Roe includes only surgical and non-surgical abortions (chemical) done at abortion facilities. It does not count the many abortions, caused by oral contraceptives, Prostaglandin, DEPO-PROVERA, IUDs, and NORPLANT. According to "Infant Homicides through Contraceptives" by Bogomir Kuhar, Ph.D., Pharmaceutical Sciences, many oral contraceptives and other contracepting systems are actually abortifacients. Kuhar estimates that from 8 to 11 million other abortions should be added to annual count of abortions in the U.S.A.

2

The Existing Pro-Life Structure

"**Whatever else it** is, the pro-life movement of the last thirty-plus years is one of the most massive and sustained expressions of citizen participation in the history of the United States." This quote is from Father Richard Neuhaus in 2009, just before his death. Before Roe v. Wade and the pro-lifers, most citizen activists were lefties and most public moral issues were described from a southpaw angle. Then why is the pro-life movement viewed as a right-wing cause? Shouldn't current public moralists like pro-lifers be called left wingers instead? What's changed? We live in strange times with curious, contemporary political alignments.

Forty five percent of respondents in a recent survey reported participating in a national protest because of abortion. Seventy five percent of all abortion issue protesters are pro-life, an unsurprising fact given that the pro-life movement is challenging rather than defending the current policy regime. All other social issues, including pornography, homosexual rights, school prayer, and sex education account for only three percent of protest activity.

"The Democratic Virtues of the Christian Right," a book by Professor Jon Shields says there are three categories of pro-life politics: deliberative, disjointed, and radical. He includes the Center for Bio-Ethical Reform and Justice for All as groups in the "deliberative" category. Those organizations have trained thousands of young people to engage in non-confrontational, pro-life persuasion on college campuses. The "disjointed" category includes a mixed bag of activities such as prayer vigils, marches and demonstrations. Shields says, the "radical" component consists of what's left of the Operation Rescue movement still focused on civil disobedience and the closing of abortion clinics.

He also decries the lack of free speech in the academic world. He describes pro-life programs at college campuses often meeting with vicious hostility, led by faculty members. Anyone in the pro-life movement has seen such hostility. It reflects the vehement opposition from pro-aborts to any civil deliberation or debate about abortion. According to Shields, this hostility is planned and organized by NARAL and Planned Parenthood.

Those anti-lifers discourage their campus affiliates from debating or even talking to pro-life students. NARAL's "Campus Kit for Pro-Choice Organizers", for example, gives this categorical instruction, "Don't waste time talking to anti-choice people." The campus organizer for Planned Parenthood told Shields that she "discourages direct debate."

The pro-life movement is a movement for change. The opposition sees it as radical change, because we want to eliminate the unlimited abortion license. The pro-abortion movement today is really the conservative movement, defending the status quo. Of course, we know the pro-aborts are not politically conservative, but I say once more that we live in strange times with curious contemporary political alignments. Pro-aborts have little to gain from engaging us in deliberative persuasion. Why should they? They have the establishment media, the courts, most politicians and academe, submissively on their side.

Although Shields categorizes three types of pro-life groups, I think there are more types of anti-abortion organizations than just three. There are many different missions in this fight against abortion. Below I will separate those different types of agencies from my perspective. There are at least five distinct categories of pro-life groups. I will list them in no particular order of importance.

The first is the legislative, lobbying and educational associations, national and state. National Right to Life (NRTL), Massachusetts Citizens for Life (from my own state) and other state affiliates of NRTL are examples. The state affiliates have many local city or regional chapters. These groups are the backbone of the pro-life movement.

The second category is the pro-life maternity homes. Such homes are unfortunately becoming rare because of the high costs of 24 hours a day, 7 days a week care for pregnant women and babies, and also because of onerous government regulations and bureaucracy. These homes provide free, warm and loving places for needy pregnant women. Visitation House, Worcester, Massachusetts, Good Counsel Homes, Hoboken, New Jersey and the Annunciation Maternity Home in Washington, D.C. are examples.

The third category is the religious pro-life organizations; e.g. the U.S. Conference of Catholic Bishops, the Southern Baptist Convention, the Pentecostal Church in America and the Eastern Orthodox Church. Each has a pro-life effort. These organizations try to use the media to press for the elimination of abortion and for abortion restrictions. They also do lobbying of politicians to the same ends. There are also various independent religious, pro-life activist groups like; the Knights of Columbus, Orthodox Christians for Life, Baptists for Life, LDS Family Services (Mormon), Episcopalians for Life, Presbyterians Pro-Life, NOEL, Lutherans for Life and others.

The fourth category is a catchall. There are many independent groups that have specific missions to preserve human life from conception to natural death. I list just a few: Priests for Life, Staten Island, New York; American Life

League, Stafford, Virginia; Pro-Life Action League, Chicago; Billboards for Life, Floyds Knobs, Indiana, Human Life International (HLI), Front Royal, Virginia; American United for Life (AUL), Washington, D.C. which defends human life by legislative and judicial efforts; Silent No More (800-707-6635), women who are recovering from past abortions and are working to stop abortions; Alliance Defense Fund, Scottsdale Arizona, legally defending pro-lifers rights, and Life Dynamics, Denton, Texas, a very aggressive pro-life research and media organization.

The fifth category is the pro-life political organizations. Groups like the Susan B. Anthony List, Arlington, Virginia, a PAC that endorses pro-life women candidates; other political action committees that support federal and state pro-life candidates financially like MCFL PAC, Boston; Life-Guard PAC, which I founded and many others. This is a very small list and many effective, pro-life organizations are missing.

3.

What Is Needed to Save Real Babies?

All of the pro-life agencies, listed in Chapter 2, try to stop abortion indirectly by educating the public about abortion or by changing legislative, judicial or electoral votes.

Professor Hadley Arkes in a "Catholic Thing" column (June 2010) wrote the following, "As we have seen over the years, the risk is to get so carried away by concerns for 'marketing' the pro-life message . . . , that the pro-lifers begin to lose their focus on the killing of an innocent being . . ."

What I propose is that we indeed not forget the "killing of an innocent being". Instead, that we non-violently and within the law concentrate our pro-life efforts with direct action at the door of the abortion mills, where those "innocent beings" are being killed. What I propose is a commingling of two, not yet mentioned types of pro-life groups; crisis pregnancy centers (CPCs) and sidewalk counseling efforts. My proposal brings pregnancy centers right next door to abortion facilities and would train volunteer sidewalk counselors to work hand-in-glove with the nearby centers. This already happens in many places in the U.S.A., but it needs to be in every killing place coast to coast. I want pro-lifers to do something positive to at least slow the wholesale slaughter of American babies.

In this scenario, the sidewalk counselor would persuade the abortion-intent woman on her way to abort to instead come to the CPC next door, hear about practical alternatives and potentially change her mind. Everything about this project will be tough. Getting the leaders. Getting the money. Getting the correct real estate proximate to the "clinic" is crucial but often difficult. Such a national effort would save lots of babies, perhaps up to ten percent of the million plus babies killed each year by abortionists. It might put some marginally profitable "clinics" out of business too.

There are two types of pro-life people necessary to operate these combination pregnancy centers and sidewalk counseling organizations (CPC Plus). Both types are most likely women and each has certain characteristics. One is the warm, loving, motherly woman wanting to help pregnant mothers and their babies while working inside a free pregnancy center. This volunteer is comfortable in a center office but not on the frontline outside an abortionist's office. The other type is the volunteer who could be motherly also but is more aggressive and knows that her efforts to speak to the abortion intent woman on her way into the abortion facility may be the last chance to save that baby from a painful death. This outside volunteer probably wishes, she could do another less stressful, pro-life job but realizes that she might be the only one who could persuade the mother and save the baby. Both types are necessary.

4.

"The powers-that-be want me to go away. My very presence in front of an abortion facility brings the nasty odor of abortion to the public's nose. Many a political, religious and business leader wants to put a clothespin on his nose to avoid what his nostrils tell him is a very bad smelling situation. Abortion happens invisibly behind antiseptic walls, allowing those community leaders to ignore this distasteful subject, as they have for 37 years. I'm not going away." Rod Murphy 2008

Saving Babies at Calvary

This is a description of the likely chronology and experience of a typical abortion client. Let's call her Jill. She is 30 years old, unmarried and lives with her boyfriend in Worcester, Massachusetts, a city of 180 thousand people. She misses a period and begins to worry that she might be pregnant. She is concerned about what a baby would mean to her relationship with her man. She then uses a home pregnancy test that confirms that she is indeed pregnant. She tells her boyfriend and it causes much consternation and argument. He is not interested in being a father and he tells her so. He uses the worn-out cliché, never really put into practice, that it is her decision, as to what should be done. Immediately thereafter, he puts pressure on her to abort the baby. She goes to her women friends for support. They make the correct sympathetic noises but do not support her having the baby. More pressure toward abortion. She calls her mother in another state. Her mother's advice is to have the abortion. Mom thinks Jill's boyfriend is a slug and will not support her and Jill will be sentenced to a very difficult life as a single mother. Still no support for the innocent baby to live, even from the baby's grandmother. No one has given her advice or support to let her pregnancy come to fruition and naturally deliver her little boy or girl.

Jill looks in the yellow pages or goes on line to see where she can get an abortion. She sees Planned Parenthood listed under abortion. She calls for an appointment and Planned Parenthood sets her up for an abortion on Friday morning at 8:30 on Pleasant Street, across the street from Problem Pregnancy. She is warned not to speak to the religious fanatics outside the abortion facility, when she arrives. On Friday, as Jill walks toward Planned Parenthood, she is met outside the "clinic" by a grandmotherly sidewalk counselor, who asks her if she needs a pregnancy test or any practical help. The counselor points out the pregnancy center across the street. The client is given some literature, showing the development of her baby at that precise moment. Jill will then decide whether she will go into the abortion facility and kill her baby or if she will go across the street and save her baby's life. That is the stark reality of life and death today at an abortion site in the U.S.A.

Now I'm going to attempt to persuade my readers to join me in this national effort by setting up their own combination CPC and sidewalk counseling effort. Isn't it time pro-lifers got angry about the taking of life right there in your own neighborhood? Isn't it time we stopped complaining about the state legislature, the Congress, the media, academia, and now President Obama? Isn't it time pro-lifers appreciated our own power and acted on it? I think so and I'm going to give you a formula on how to do just that. Each of you has the opportunity, the responsibility, yes, and the sacred duty of saving some of the millions of abortions per year or hundreds of thousands of abortions per day. There are over 31 hundred babies killed annually at our local Planned Parenthood. Find out how many babies are being slaughtered in your city's abortion mills each year. In the Appendix of this book you will find a list of all the abortion facilities in the fifty states. We often hear from well-meaning folks, that we need only do our best. Just make sure you try. Bull! We are fighting a horrendous evil. I believe God expects us to be successful. He expects us to win. Just trying isn't enough. We must save some of those 35 hundred innocent babies chopped up every day. That requires a defense and an offense. It requires people to do something now! St. John states, "Let us love, not in word or speech, but in truth and action". How are we to do that?

Let me tell you. I started in the pro-life movement as a young husband and father before Roe v. Wade. I have lived the whole history of abortion from when it was an abhorrent crime to now, where it has become almost a feminist sacrament. I've seen and lived all the pro-life responses to abortion. I was a local pro-life chapter chairman and I was a Massachusetts Citizens for Life state board director in the seventies and eighties. I have fought many battles in the political arena, trying to get pro-lifers elected and pro-aborts retired. Lately, however I have become very disillusioned and weary with politics. I've been arrested many times with Operation Rescue, blockading abortion facilities in the eighties and nineties. But my most effective, pro-life action has been with crisis pregnancy centers. Those of us, frustrated with the usual pro-life efforts, get great satisfaction from snatching just one real baby away from the abortionist's curette.

In 1982 Problem Pregnancy, a pregnancy resource center in Worcester, Massachusetts, was founded. I've been the director and CEO most of the time since then. We are one of about two thousand crisis pregnancy centers in the U.S., working to save babies, one stopped abortion at a time. In order to effectively save babies constantly every day from the abortionist, a strategic CPC location next door or very close to the abortion facility is necessary. That address will become the focus of most of the pro-life effort in your city, because you will be saving real baby boys and girls. Taking money away from the evil abortionists is a secondary benefit.

If there is anything that the reader should take from this book, it would be my hope that my readers not allow another local mother to pay a stranger $650 to rip the arms and legs off her precious, pre-born daughter or son, and then throw her offspring into the medical garbage. Without a frontline crisis pregnancy center competing for babies' lives, Planned Parenthood or other abortionist will slaughter every one of the 35 hundred American pre-borns, scheduled for abortion every day. Action is necessary. If there is no frontline free pregnancy center, offering alternatives near the local abortionist in your city, start one. That new frontline pregnancy center must be augmented with an aggressive sidewalk counseling effort.

In the U.S.A. each year almost a million pregnant women and adolescents visit CPCs. There are over 40 thousand volunteers working at those free pregnancy centers. Twenty-nine of every thirty people, working at such pro-life pregnancy centers, are volunteers.

Problem Pregnancy is the oldest and the most successful frontline pregnancy center in Massachusetts. Unfortunately we have not vanquished the abortionists in Worcester. They kill about 31 hundred babies and we save over two hundred each year. We have a lot further to go, but we fight for each life on the abortion frontline. So, I am going to describe in this book a model for you to use in setting up a pregnancy resource center with a sidewalk counseling program. We actually save babies. You can and should save babies too!

Problem Pregnancy, now in its 28th year, has always been located next door to Planned Parenthood's abortion facility. The abortionists have had three different Worcester locations and we have followed them each time. We had already moved into a former doctor's office across the street, before they finished their latest $5 million downtown fortress.

Pro-life pregnancy centers are the new face of an old movement: kind and nonjudgmental, but we are the Delta Forces in the abortion wars, fighting our battles, one woman's conscience at a time. Our volunteers are no different from you. We are weak reeds and need lots of help from our prayer-answering God. We know that saving babies in the wombs of mothers on their way into an abortion mill requires that we physically be there at that abortion facility. In Worcester our volunteers pray and sidewalk counsel at Planned Parenthood's front and back door four days a week when surgical abortions and medical abortions are committed. Those volunteers with great difficulty bring wavering clients to our adjacent office. We have been doing that for 28 years. In order for the abortion minded mother to have her so-called choice, she needs to hear the truth.

In my city, it has fallen upon us, pro-life, Christian laypeople to tell the truth about abortion because no one else is doing it. Did Christ tell His disciples to stay in their churches and talk to each other about the Gospel or didn't He say to go out and preach the Gospel and the truth to the world? We must take the truth to our neighbors in Worcester and you, readers, must do it in your city, to the needy pregnant women, who think that abortion is their only answer.

The truth: 15 thousand babies will perish this year at the three Planned Parenthood abortion mills in my state. How many in your state? Find out. The truth: Many women are killed or grievously injured by abortions at supposedly safe clinics. The truth: Many other women will have mental problems throughout their lives, caused by an abortion. The truth: medical studies show that women, who have had an abortion, have a much higher incidence of breast cancer. Another truth, now proven by 17 studies, confirms that abortion causes very premature birth in the previously aborted woman's next pregnancy. And the latest 2010 truth: a new study conducted by researchers at the University of Manitoba found that women who have had abortions are four times more likely to abuse drugs and alcohol as those who delivered their babies. Those truths are not known by most Americans. You must tell those truths to the confused, pregnant woman carrying her innocent but condemned baby in your city. We do that in Worcester. Shouldn't you be ashamed that thousands of babies are being killed in your city? Shouldn't you get damn angry and shouldn't you do something about that carnage just down the street from you?

A 1994 Reader Digest article by Mary Cunningham Agee reported that 91 percent of women surveyed in post-abortion interviews stated that they would have carried their child to term, if support had been there. Those of us taking on this critical volunteer job must understand that often a woman will abort her child because she thinks her problems will be solved. But you must try to discover her truth — the real reasons she is considering abortion. It often isn't her pregnancy that is the real problem but ancillary things that are overwhelming her. Things like an overdue telephone bill, college tuition bill, or a broken-down car that needs repairs. The kind of things that money can cure. Raising money for your CPC will provide that aid for mothers and their babies.

When a new pregnancy center is started, I suggest that it be all-volunteer and that no one get paid. The reason obviously is that such a model cuts the cost of operation down to a minimum and allows a shoestring operation to begin. Your mission should be to provide anything that a woman needs, the lack of which is causing her to consider abortion. She will be concerned about things, such as housing, unpaid bills, legal help, immigration help, maternity care, psychological or spiritual counseling, referrals for adoption, baby cribs, maternity clothes or many other needs. We've saved babies by making overdue car payments and more than once we have paid for a wedding with reception, so that the baby would live. We have bought airline tickets to Africa and South America so an abortion-pressured client could go home to her family instead of aborting her baby. No life should end because of money.

If you provide that practical help, the need for abortion is lessened and the baby often lives; e.g. if a baby will die, because a client has no apartment, then you must pay for an apartment. Parents and boyfriends often threaten that unless our client has an abortion, she will be evicted from their home. By taking responsibility for that kind of real life problems, we really do provide a choice and an alternative to abortion. I strongly suggest your CPC do the same.

There has never been a situation, when we needed to save a baby by helping a mother, and we didn't have the necessary funds. God is very generous and He has lots of hundred dollar bills. Nine years ago we bought a $25 thousand ultrasound. The building, we just bought across the street from the abortionists, cost almost a half million dollars. We always get what is needed. We continually pay expensive and on-going client rents, so babies may live. Donors love to contribute to an effective organization. If you save babies, you will attract donors. God has provided for us for 28 years. He will for you also. Be not afraid! You must have faith in God and you must act!

Problem Pregnancy Inc. started in 1982 with about 20 pro-lifers and a pro-bono lawyer when Planned Parenthood expanded into our city. If an abortionist is operating without pro-life competition, then a frontline CPC is needed in your city. You can do it. Plan it. Organize the volunteers and find the location very close to the abortionist. Pastor Susan Lynch, a friend and former Assembly of God pastor uses an expression that I have picked up, "Act with holy boldness". In other words, step out in faith and do it!

Willie Sutton, the notorious bank robber was asked once why he robbed banks. He answered because that's where the money is. In the same vein, we need to be located near the abortionists, because that's where babies are killed. The bible asks us to be as shrewd as serpents and as innocent as doves. We must use our intelligence. As I have said, we must not just try; we must succeed in saving babies.

There may be very good pro-life counseling centers in your city. They have probably been helping pregnant women for years. Please don't think that I am disparaging that work. Problem Pregnancy has a satellite office in Athol, Massachusetts, a small working class city near the New Hampshire border. Because that office is not near an abortion mill, our client rate there is low and so is our baby-save rate but it still does good work, helping mothers and babies. The same is true with other non-frontline centers. The target market for the two types of CPCs is different. From my experience, the pregnancy centers not located near an abortion facility get clients, who ordinarily don't really want an abortion. Otherwise those clients would be at the abortion "clinic". They need affirming of their pro-life decision and they usually are very needy of material things. We call them "wannabe moms". However frontline CPCs locate their offices adjacent to abortion facilities and are aggressive with sidewalk counselors, right outside the abortion mill. They have a very different mandate. The policy at these centers is to save the baby's life, often at the very last possible moment and then try to straighten out the mother's life, if possible.

These centers are often Roman Catholic oriented, but independent of the Church. The client market for frontline centers is very different from the non-frontline type. The woman on her way into Planned Parenthood to destroy her child is the target for frontline CPCs. This category of center gets their client in absolute extremis. They are the baby's last resort. The two types of CPCs are not competitors. They complement each other. The client base is different. All types of centers should work together to help women and save babies.

Pregnancy centers need to be right in the face of the abortion facility. More specifically unless the location of the center is within the vision of the abortionist's clients, driving or walking in, the center will not get the intended, numerous baby-saves. Is there any magic bullet to stop this holocaust? Yes... you are that magic bullet. With the right facility and in the right location, pro-lifers can change the hearts of many abortion minded mothers. Lay counselors need to be trained but do not need to be professionals. Pregnancy centers need women, who are nurses, teachers, blue collar workers, business people, retired folks and especially mothers who understand pregnancy and life best of all.

Much of the pro-life movement remains focused on changing laws and tightening restrictions on abortions, one by one, state by state. But pregnancy centers talk of changing minds and hearts. They are part of a new strategy that is more feminine, more personal and more pastoral. CPC personnel hear so often from clients, who have had previous abortions and now know the truth, "No one told me. If only someone had explained it to me and talked to me. I would not have aborted my child." You must be that someone for her to talk to in your own city!

My idea, my dream is a national effort to put a CPC with sidewalk counseling next door to every American abortion facility. It will be a big job. If we had such a pro-life pregnancy center next door to every American abortion site and if each center could save ten percent of the endangered babies, then nationally, hundreds of thousands of condemned babies would be saved. And hundreds of thousands of mothers would not be sentenced to a lifetime of regret and potential bad medical side effects. The time is now. The place is there in your neighborhood. The prize is great! We have a job to do and how historic a job it is. So stop dithering! Let's together do something for those endangered babies and for God. Why can't we put pregnancy centers next door to abortionists all over America? Let's intervene with that mother in your city, who would have hired that stranger to crush the head of her baby. Shouldn't we save some of those thirty five hundred babies scheduled to be destroyed today? I say yes! What say you?

5.

Abortion History and Background

In 1973, the U.S. Supreme Court made a decision that produced the most unrestricted abortion law in the world. That decision is called Roe v Wade. At the time, America was a relatively pro-life country. That decision began the rockslide of American morality. Abortion is overwhelming in its disintegration of all components of a civil society. The number of abortions done legally since the 1973 Roe v. Wade U.S. Supreme Court decision is estimated to be 52 million*, as of 2009. Our current population (2009) estimate is 303 million people. That means that in 36 years, Americans have aborted 16% of its population. Much of that missing population, if it had not been destroyed, would be paying taxes and Social Security and helping to keep our economy stable today in this recession.

---

* Counting the number of abortions is complicated. The 1.2 million abortions per year and the 52 million abortions since Roe include only surgical and non-surgical abortions (chemical) done at abortion facilities. It does not count the many abortions, caused by oral contraceptives, Prostaglandin, Depo-Provera, IUDs, and Norplant. According to "Infant Homicides through Contraceptives" by Bogomir Kuhar, Ph.D., Pharmaceutical Sciences, many oral contraceptives and other contracepting systems are actually abortifacients. Kuhar estimates that from 8 to 11 million other abortions should be added to the annual count of abortions in the U.S.A.

In recent years, the abortion rate has decreased. Some of that decrease should be credited to the years of different pro-life organizations working to change the public's mind on abortion. But much of the decrease comes as a result of demographics. There are simply fewer women of child-bearing age. The Centers for Disease Control, using the census numbers, reports that the birth rate is dropping, as the increasing life span of Americans results in a smaller proportion of women of child childbearing age. In other words, we have too many old farts, like Rod Murphy and not enough fertile mothers having babies. Where did those young women go? Do you think it could it have anything to do with the Roe v. Wade decision 37 years ago?

Those Roe justices and other subsequent courts, Houdini-like, smoked out a formerly hidden-away constitutional right to abortion for any reason and at any time during pregnancy. Yet, the general public remains almost uniformly uninform-ed about what Roe v. Wade and its companion decision, Doe v. Bolton means and what would happen, if it were overturned. Recent polls have found that, while 65 percent of Americans said they are familiar with Roe, only 29 percent could select an accurate description of the ruling. Another national poll of registered voters attempted to measure the public's knowledge about Roe. Respondents were asked a generic question about whether or not they wanted Roe overturned. 55 percent said "no," and only 34 percent supported overturning Roe. But after an explanation was given as to what Roe means—that it prohibits states from limiting abortion during the first six months of pregnancy, the share that opposed reversing Roe dropped seven points to 48 percent. Meanwhile, the portion that supported overturning Roe jumped nine points, to 43 percent, a 16-point swing.

Some pro-lifers seem to have accepted a notion that their ultimate goal is the reversal of Roe v. Wade. Just get one more pro-life justice on the Supreme Court, they say, then Roe will be overturned and abortion will be a thing of the past.

In June of 2010 former Solicitor General Walter Dellinger, no friend of endangered unborn babies, predicted that the Supreme Court would eventually overturn Roe v. Wade. The method, he said, will be replacing Justice Anthony Kennedy with a pro-life judge. Most abortion advocates won't admit that the day is coming when that infamous decision will be struck down and states may then be able to offer legal protection for women and unborn children.

The truth is that Roe's reversal would not end the abortion wars. Rather, it would mark the beginning of another battle, to which the last 37 years has been just the prologue. The day after Roe's reversal, abortion policy would revert to the states and that would begin another hot political battle. Thank God, I will be gone.

In the aftermath of Roe's demise (that is sure to come), some states would ban or severely restrict abortion. States, mostly along the two coasts, would most likely pass laws guaranteeing the same access to abortion as would be present at the time of Roe's end. Only a minority of states would vote a total abortion ban. The rest would probably battle it out for many years. Our nation's fundamental commitment to the right to life shows up in both the second paragraph of the Declaration of Independence and the 14th Amendment to the U.S. Constitution (No state shall "deprive any person of life, liberty, or property without due process of law").

Does this mean overturning Roe v. Wade should not remain a top priority for pro-lifers? No, scrapping Roe is important, because it would allow a real discussion about abortion to take place. We can win that argument.

6.

What is a Crisis Pregnancy Center?

Crisis pregnancy centers (CPCs) are an absolutely necessary facet of the pro-life movement. CPCs provide alternatives to abortion. Sometimes such centers are just a few volunteers and sometimes they are larger, some with multiple locations. CPCs or as they are also called pregnancy centers do invaluable work, saving the lives of babies and helping mothers to avoid making a huge moral error.

Many women clients do not want an abortion and need help and advice on how to be successful as a single mother. Others have decided to abort and are coming to us for many different reasons, sometimes by mistake and sometimes hoping someone will talk them out of it. Many simply are ambivalent about what to do. CPCs help all the different categories of clients, no matter what their initial intent. Many clients tell counselors that they have no choice and they must have an abortion. Yet many of those will change their minds, when given the facts in a loving, supportive environment.

In the beginning of the crisis pregnancy center movement, the typical center consisted of a few volunteers, some diapers and baby clothes and an offer of a free pregnancy test. There are still some of these small centers but many of today's centers have grown and now reach an increasingly demand-ing and discriminating clientele.

The National Right to Life Educational Trust Fund conducted a national CPC survey in 1999 and found a wide array of services and institutional arrangements. Those data, although somewhat out of date, will help the reader under-stand about the modern CPC. Thirty-four states were counted, representing CPCs of various sizes, budgets, and situations. Many of the CPCs still had the traditional arrangement—small centers with modest budgets in small communities staffed by volunteers. But an increasing number consisted of large scale operations, with at least some paid professional staff, medical, social services, and budgets over $100 thousand. Ninety-six of the hundred surveyed centers operated at least partially with volunteers.

The survey discovered that some CPCs also relied upon paid staff as leaders. About half had at least one paid full-time employee, while two-thirds reported paid part-time employees. Almost universally, training for volunteers was provided at CPCs according to the survey. The study reported that the increasing presence of staff with medical or social work training was benefiting the centers. An average of two medically trained workers and at least one staffer trained in social work were on a typical larger CPC staff, according to the survey. Bringing in medical services and professional personnel shows the maturing of the CPC movement.

The easily purchased home pregnancy test kits have reduced the draw of the CPCs' free pregnancy test offer. The financially secure, career-oriented woman is especially difficult to get into our centers. Sometimes a free ultrasound scan will entice them. Heartbeat International is a national association of CPC members. Many of Heartbeat's affiliates offer ultrasound. More CPCs are in the process of adding the scanners, according to Beth Diemert of Heartbeat. She is very positive about the impact of ultrasound. She says that, after seeing their child on the ultrasound screen, 60 to 90 percent of clients will change their minds and decide not to abort.

Ultrasound equipment is expensive and so are sonographers, even though those services are often volunteered. A good used ultrasound machine runs over $20 thousand. In order to upgrade to ultrasound, pregnancy centers must raise more funds for their budgets. National Right to Life's survey shows increasing numbers of CPCs with yearly outlays in six figures. One third of their 1999 surveyed centers reported an annual budget in excess of $100 thousand, with one sixth having budgets in excess of $200 thousand. Very few centers had budgets of $25 thousand or less. Despite the fact that they do not charge for their services, many CPCs think that they must add ultrasound to compete with the abortion "clinics." The survey found that free pregnancy tests, baby clothes, diapers and maternity clothes were offered by nearly every center. Other services offered were mediation with parent(s) or with the client's boyfriend, adoption referrals, parenting classes, educational assistance, birthing classes, financial counseling, and legal assistance. While medical referrals were common, a few centers even went so far as to cover costs of prenatal care, delivery, and postnatal care in some cases. We do even more in Worcester!

Pregnancy resource centers or crisis pregnancy centers have been around since 1968, even before Roe v Wade. After Roe, the social context of an unmarried woman's pregnancy became charged with pressure to abort and abortion is now the norm in such situations. CPCs are the Christian response to that phenomenon. I repeat there are more than two thousand of these agencies in the U.S.A. These centers offer alternatives to abortion to pregnant mothers: counseling, pregnancy tests, material aid, ultrasound scans, lots of love and other practical help. A few examples of pregnancy resource centers are Problem Pregnancy, Worcester, Massachusetts; Women's Center, Chicago; Emergency Mother Care (EMC); Bronx, New York and Pregnancy Care Center, Fort Pierce, Florida.

Naming Your CPC

Words and names are important as to how we are perceived. The name of a new CPC should be neutral sounding and attractive to women. In Worcester, we named our organization Problem Pregnancy, which got immediately confused with Planned Parenthood. This PP confusion has brought many clients into our office and helped many babies to be saved from painful death. Planned Parenthood sued Problem Pregnancy during our early years, because we were using our own initials (PP) on our office door. Obviously, the initials are the same as Planned Parenthood's. Both organizations were in the same large downtown Worcester office building and on the same floor. We had "corridor counselors" at the elevator doors. Our counselors were intervening with abortion intent mothers, bringing them to our PP office and not to the bad guys' PP office, further down the corridor.

We were having great baby-saving success and Planned Parenthood was furious and sued us. A Massachusetts Superior Court judge (Elbert Tuttle) ruled in Planned Parenthood's favor and ordered Problem Pregnancy to put a Crucifix on our front door near our PP sign. Problem Pregnancy is not a Catholic outfit. We are a non-sectarian group yet the ruling forced not just a cross, but a Roman Catholic Crucifix with the Corpus of the hanging and suffering Jesus. This decision had many observers seeing glimpses of the thirties and forties in Germany, with Jews forced by the Nazis to wear Stars of David on their clothing. The whole matter was memorialized and recorded by the sainted Congressman Henry Hyde in the U.S. Congressional Record.

I'm working with a group of great and creative pro-lifers to open a new CPC in Springfield, Massachusetts. Their center is called the New Women's Center (NWC). What do you think when you first hear that name? My first thought is that such a center would be a New Age, feminist, crunchy bunch of lesbians, providing abortions, condoms and man-hating advice. The clients with abortion appointments could easily mistake NWC for an abortion mill. Just what we want, eh? All abortionists warn their clients with abortion appointments to avoid pro-lifers and Christians on the way to abort. NWC's name and whole presentation is neutral and overcomes that cautionary advice so it will not frighten the potential baby-saves away.

The purpose of a CPC is to save babies and help mothers, not to save mothers' souls (more about this later) therefore the name of the organization should be strategic (Strategy—a plan of action designed to achieve a particular goal.) By strategic I mean that, like the location, like the signs out front, like the sidewalk counselors working the abortion facility's front door, the name also should help to further the mission. Names like "Bethany Christian Center," "Grace for Babies Ministry, "Breath of Life Center" or the "St. Teresa Family Center" are wrong and telegraph our pro-life intentions to women—the same women that were told to avoid the crazy pro-lifers, when they reach the abortion facility. We need tactics not doctrines.

The same idea about tactics needs to be pursued inside the CPC and outside with the sidewalk counselors. No religious tracts, holy pictures, rosary beads, newborn baby pictures, cutesy-poo toys, teddy bears, cribs or car seats, etc. should be visible when the clients walk into the office.

Magazines in the waiting room should be the usual secular junk that women read, not Catholic World Report or Christianity Today. The attitude of the receptionist/coun-selor should be more friendly and professional and less maternal. Every action done by pro-lifers should respond to the hope and the prayer that this mother will be persuaded to change her mind from abortion to life for her baby. Outside on the sidewalk, designated counselors should pray of course but not overtly. Of course, sidewalk counselors especially need God's help and should ask for it all the time but not openly.

There are different opinions on this. Some pro-lifers think that some clients are unknowingly starved for God. They think that offering a set of rosary beads or a religious tract will be welcomed and a dialogue will open up and perhaps save a baby.

* * *

Problem Pregnancy has a Commitment of Care that we adapted from the Heartbeat International's CPC code. It is printed with calligraphy-like letters, framed and proudly hung in an easily seen spot on the office wall. Here are the individual points.

1.   Clients of PPW are served free and without regard to age, race, income, nationality, religious affiliation, disability or other arbitrary circumstances.

2.   Clients of PPW are not required to listen to religious or church information without giving full consent and without any quid pro quo about possible withheld services.

3.   Clients of PPW are treated with kindness, compassion and in a caring manner and always receive honest and open answers.

4.   Client services are distributed and administered in accordance with all applicable laws.

5. Client information is held in strict and absolute confidence. Client information is only disclosed as required by law and when necessary to protect the client or others against imminent harm.

6. Clients of PPW receive accurate information about pregnancy, fetal development, lifestyle issues, and related concerns.

7. PPW does not offer, recommend or refer for abortions or abortifacients, but is committed to offering accurate information about abortion procedures and risks.

8. All staff and volunteers of PPW receive proper training to uphold these standards.

Social Entrepreneurship

The phrase "social entrepreneur" is a relatively new term but I like it. Although it now has a name, it is not a new idea. It describes what really happens, when a person or a group finds a social need and founds an organization to fill that need. Very much like a small business entrepreneur, who sees an opportunity to make money, filling an unfulfilled, mercantile need.

Many non-profits are started by people with wonderful dreams, which they are able to sell to donors. The really hard part of implementing the dream begins then. Charisma has to be replaced by hard nosed management skills like setting up the legal structures and procedures, planning, recruiting the right staff, monitoring, managing the enterprise and in our case helping women and saving babies. Maybe it's time business schools had courses for social entrepreneurs that cover all the skills needed to make dreams come true?

I have been part of many of these social entrepreneurial beginnings. As I wrote above, I have been involved with pregnancy center start-ups. I also was a founding board member of a maternity home start-up. My working life intersects with my life as a believing Catholic. I am often asked how I got so involved in fighting abortion. My answer is long and it involves the influence of my parents and the nuns from grammar school. At the end of my answer I always encourage the questioner and others to volunteer to save babies because of the combined blessings that come to the client, to the volunteer and to the organization. Many good things come from fighting abortion.

Using myself as an example, I would tell the questioner that I am an entrepreneur. I currently own more than one business and have started many others. The things I have learned from business are put to work in my volunteer activities to the betterment of both. The things, I have learned as a volunteer leader in the pro-life movement, have helped my business in many ways also. This is called synergism. God works with us in our efforts to do His will and perform good works. He has been with me, leading me throughout my life; family, charitable and business.

All entrepreneurs are creative people and some are also pro-life. If we could recruit those pro-life entrepreneurs to put their efforts into starting CPCs, they would be able to find imaginative solutions to start-up problems. Those folks are usually ambitious and persistent, two traits needed for success. Hands-on experienced people do much better than social worker types in getting results. Business oriented volunteers need incentives. Ordinarily those incentives would be profits, earned through business success but in our plan, the incentive would come from Christian duty, love of God, concern for needy people but mostly because the social entrepreneur could reduce the number of babies, dying by the thousands at American aboratoriums. The kind of social entrepreneur I am thinking about could take an old, underperforming CPC, move it next to an abortion "clinic," change some operating methods and turn it into a baby-saving, mother-helping success. These folks have skills in leadership and in the recruitment of performance oriented volunteers. They have passion, are often visionaries and are very practical. I hope and pray they will be the leaders of this new task force.

Every pregnancy resource center needs an accepted leader. This leader, along with a board of directors and much help from other volunteers, provides the direction of the center. He or she should wake up every morning, thinking about how his center can be improved, so that it saves more babies and helps more mothers.

CPC Counseling

Free pro-life pregnancy centers, also called crisis pregnancy centers or pregnancy resource centers, aid women before, during and after pregnancy. My plan would have a CPC specialize in helping at the point of decision, when abortion is the client's chosen option. Pregnancy tests are the most frequent requests by clients. 50 percent of women tested will prove to be pregnant at CPCs. The correct attitude of the center counselor should be that she will provide anything for the pregnant client, the lack of which is causing the client to consider abortion. The counselor should visualize the abortion minded client after her baby is born and work toward that positive vision. Problem Pregnancy of Worcester, Inc., the CPC for which I am the director, sees women and girls from 13 to 35 years old, most of them unmarried. Our counselors are all volunteers and most are trained veterans, who know how to handle anxious women.

Any new CPC, like Springfield, Massachusetts' "New Women's Center" (NWC) mentioned above, should set up a training program for the new counselors. Perhaps an existing CPC could provide the training. Problem Pregnancy has done that for other new pregnancy centers and will do it for NWC. What a CPC counselor does is called crisis intervention counseling.

Listening is probably the most important thing that a CPC counselor can do. First it allows a client to vent her concerns, emotions, her panic and sometimes her anger. Second, it allows the counselor to discover by asking questions whether or not the pregnant client is considering abortion. If she is considering abortion, the counselor, by listening and asking the right questions, will try to ascertain what are the client's ancillary problems that might be pushing her towards abortion. Sometimes listening calls for what seems to be an unnatural silence on the counselor's part. That silence often will be understood by the client to mean that her counselor is concentrating on her. Sometimes that silence causes the client to open up even more to fill the void. That openness can give the counselor the key to saving the baby, if the client feels sympathy coming from her counselor.

The counselor must be nonjudgmental in dealing with clients who are often difficult and not easy to love. But love them, we must. After listening to the client's concerns, the counselor usually has achieved a certain rapport with her client. Then she must provide the facts of abortion. Using fetal models, to show the development of the client's baby, at that moment, is a powerful way to give her the facts. There are many other ways also. The client will need these facts in order to make an informed decision. The bonding with that friendly counselor grows stronger because the client feels she is not being judged.

Confidentiality is almost absolute and the client must know that anything she tells the CPC and its counselor will remain private. Child abuse or threats of suicide are two exceptions to that confidentiality.

The counselor must believe that her intervention will be advantageous to her client. The counselor should know whatever the final result; her effort will end up helping the client today or in the future.

There are three types of clients that are seen by pregnancy centers. The easiest to handle are the clients, who are morally opposed to abortion and need some material aid and a pregnancy test. The second type of woman will arrive leaning toward an abortion, but will be ambivalent because of religious concerns or perhaps a relative had influenced her toward allowing her baby to live. We will have mostly success with that type of client and her baby will be usually saved, but we lose some of those to abortion also despite good counseling.

For Problem Pregnancy, the clients most desired are also the most difficult. They are those clients with abortion appointments across the street. Often a sidewalk counselor has intervened and one of those clients is brought to the center. Another version of this type of difficult client will have mistakenly come in thinking the pregnancy center is an abortion "clinic." If you locate very near an abortion facility, you will get many of this type. We call them "Holy Spirit" clients, because we think there is continuous divine intervention, helped by our prayer. These women initially do not want to hear any alternatives. They think they have no other choice but abortion. We persevere and often are successful in saving babies.

There are at least five reasons a woman will give as to why she "needs" an abortion: her physical condition or health; her relationship with her boyfriend (almost never a husband); her relationship with her parents; her social situation such as living arrangements, finances and school; and "Is it really a baby?" is the last reason. There are many ways to handle each of these reasons, so that the baby lives.

* * *

There are many issues not covered in this short description of pregnancy counseling. Things like contraception, adoption, politics, bringing order to clients' chaotic lives, saving souls, sexually active teens, STDs, etc. I'm not going to get into details of those in this book. Some ideas in this book were gleaned from the CPC manuals* listed below.

Understanding Abortion Methods and Complications

In order to counsel abortion intent or abortion ambivalent pregnant women, we must understand what pregnancy is. Pregnancy is the process that begins with the man's sperm penetrating a woman's oocyte (egg). A human baby is thereby conceived. Nine months later that baby will enter our world from the womb. Most people would agree that *Fertilization* of the woman's egg by the man's sperm is the beginning of pregnancy. They are correct.

Planned Parenthood and others, having nefarious purposes in mind, state that *Implantation* (the attachment of the baby to the lining of his mother's uterus) is the beginning

---

* "Introduction to Pregnancy Counseling" Sr. Paula Vandegaer, S.S.S. published by International Life Services 1999
"Problem Pregnancy Office Guidelines" Problem Pregnancy Worcester, Massachusetts 2002
"Equipped to Serve" Cynthia Phikill and Suzanne Walsh Frontlines Publishing 1997

of pregnancy. Pro-lifers think that anything that interrupts that implantation should be called an abortifacient or an agent that causes abortion. Things like an abortionist, the contraceptive pill, the IUD, Norplant, Depo-Provera, etc. are such agents of abortion.

We also must understand and pass on to clients the abortionist's methods, the potential abortion risks and the potential complications to the client. The following very disturbing information about actual abortion methods comes from "Equipped to Serve" Cynthia Phikill and Suzanne Walsh published by Frontlines Publishing, 1997 and the "Pro Life Reference Journal," published by Massachusetts Citizens for Life in 2001.

Types of Abortions

First Trimester (1-14 weeks)

1. *Suction Curettage*—The abortionist dilates (opens) the cervix with mechanical dilators or laminaria (a porous substance that is typically inserted a day before the abortion). Overnight the laminaria gradually dilates the cervix by soaking up fluid. The day of the abortion the abortionist attaches tubing to a suction machine, and inserts the tubing into the uterus. The suction created by the vacuum pulls the unborn baby's body apart and detaches the

placenta from the wall of the uterus, sucking the fetal parts and placenta into a collection bottle.

2. *Dilation and Curettage* (D&C or sharp curettage) -This method as not as common anymore for abortions, because it requires more dilation and more time, and is considered less safe than suction curettage for the mother. The cervix is dilated, and a curette, or loop-shaped knife, is inserted into the uterus to cut apart the unborn baby and scrape the uterine lining to detach the placenta. All body parts and membranes are then scraped out of the mother's body.

Second Trimester (13-26 weeks)

1. *Dilation and Evacuation* (D&E) At this point in pregnancy, the unborn baby's body is too large to be broken up by suction, and it will not pass through the tubing. The cervix needs to be dilated more than in the first trimester abortion, and this is usually accomplished by inserting laminaria a day or two before the abortion. The abortionist then dismembers the body parts. The skull is crushed and the spine is broken to facilitate removal.

2. *Saline, Prostaglandin, and Urea Installation* These methods, more common during the 1970s and 1980s, are rarely used now, according the Centers for Disease Control (CDC), which reported that they accounted for only 0.7% or approximately 11,200 of all reported abortions in 1991.

In a *saline abortion,* the abortionist injects a concentrated salt solution through the mother's abdomen into the amniotic sac surrounding the baby. The fetus absorbs the solution, which causes burning, hemorrhage, edema, shock, and eventually death. The saline also causes the uterus to contract and expel the baby.

Prostaglandin abortions are performed by injecting a prostaglandin hormone into the amniotic sac. The hormone stimulates uterine contractions to expel the fetus, who has usually died, although a 1978 study showed that up to 7% of babies, aborted with prostaglandins, showed signs of life.

Urea abortions are similar to saline abortions but are not as effective. They are thought to have fewer complications for the mother. Urea infusion is more commonly combined with later-term D&E abortions to soften fetal tissues for easier safer and less painful removal for the mother.

Second and Third Trimester

1. *Dilation and Extraction (D&X) or Partial Birth Abortion*

Congressional action in 1996 brought to light yet another procedure for aborting late-term babies. This technique, called D&X abortion, does not dismember the fetus; rather, the fetus is delivered intact, `without infusions. As described and performed abortion doctor Martin Haskell, D&X

abortions take three days to complete. In the first two days, the woman's cervix is dilated with laminaria in two or more sessions, with medication given for cramping. On the day of the procedure, the laminaria are removed, and the patient is injected with Pitocin to induce contractions. The abortion doctor next determines the fetus' orientation in the uterus through ultrasound, and locates the legs. Grasping a leg with a large forceps, he then pulls the leg into the vagina and delivers the baby (live) up to the baby's head with his hands. Next the abortionist slides his hand up the baby's back and hooks his fingers over the shoulders of the baby. Then a pair of scissors is inserted into the base of the skull to create an opening. Removing the scissors, he inserts a suction catheter into the opening and suctions out the skull contents. Minus its brains, the skull decompresses, and is easy to remove. Finally, the abortionist removes the placenta with forceps and scrapes the uterine walls. This method is now outlawed.

Physical Risks of Risks of Abortion

First Trimester

Cervical tearing and laceration from the instruments and perforation of the uterus by instruments are physical risks of abortion. May require major surgery, including hysterectomy. Scarring of the uterine lining by suction tubing, curettes and other instruments are also physical risks of abortion.. Infections, local and systemic (sepsis) are physical risks of abortion too. Hemorrhage and shock, especially if the uterine wall is torn are likely. And these are risks: anesthesia toxicity from both general or local anesthesia, resulting in convulsions; cardio-respiratory arrest, and in extreme cases, death; general anesthesia in abortion has a two to four times greater risk of death than local anesthesia; retained tissue, indicated by cramping, heavy bleeding and infection; post-abortal syndrome, referring to an enlarged, tender and soft uterus retaining blood clots; failure to recognize an ectopic pregnancy which could lead to the rupture of a fallopian tube and hemorrhage and resulting infertility or death, if treatment is not provided in time.

Second Trimester

Infusion methods

All of the following are risks from abortions: "Failed Abortion," also known as "live birth"; retained tissue, including the placenta. uterine rupture, with resulting severe pain and blood loss which may require major surgery, including hysterectomy; cervical laceration, perforation, heavy bleeding or hemorrhage, and infection.

Dilation and Evacuation

All of the following are risks from abortions: trapped fetal parts, leading to possible damage to the uterus and nearby organs, such as the bowel and bladder; laceration and perforation of the uterus and/or cervix by fetal parts and/or the larger instruments used in these midterm abortions; general risk of hemorrhage.

* * *

Complications from Abortions

How often do complications and death occur? Getting accurate statistics on abortion morbidity (complications) and mortality (death) rates is difficult. The rates are generally accepted as underreported. Reporting on abortions is strictly voluntary in most states, and both the CDC and the Alan Guttmacher Institute (a Planned Parenthood ally) acknowledge a significant undercount in their statistics on the number of abortions performed. The rate of major complications resulting from abortion is usually reported around 2 percent. The risk of complications rises as a pregnancy progresses. In many cases, abortionists may not even know that complications occur, because many women do not contact them, if they experience problems. Another reality, as we know at Problem Pregnancy, is many women fail to show up for follow-up appointments.

The CDC reports that between 1979 and 1986 almost 5 percent of maternal deaths were due to abortion, including those deaths involving spontaneous abortions (miscarriages). The leading causes of death from abortion, during 1979-1986, were hemorrhage from uterine bleeding, generalized infection, and blood clots in the lungs. However, many abortion-related deaths are disguised and not listed as such. Complications of childbirth and/or some other factors, caused by the abortion but not mentioned, are often listed as the cause.

To further illustrate the problem, Surgeon General C. Everett Koop, in his 1989 letter to President Ronald Reagan, explained that the lack of scientifically sound studies made it impossible to "provide conclusive data about the health effects of abortion on women" and wrote that complications are difficult to quantify for two reasons: first because abortions are done in free-standing "clinics," where records, which might have been helpful in this regard, are missing. Second, when compared with the number of abortions performed annually, 50 percent of women, who have had an abortion, apparently deny having one. Therefore, according to Koop, the statistics are almost useless.

Operating a CPC

Retail experts know that the internal and external appearance of a store is important in getting customers inside. Pregnancy resource centers should pick up on this savvy business practice. Our offices should be inviting, safe, friendly, well lighted and bright. Are your clients personally welcomed as they come in the front door? Is the reception area and waiting room brightly lit? Does the appearance look orderly and well decorated? A CPC should be a working office with staff, computers, phones ringing (I hope), private counseling rooms, a coffee pot and a professional appearance.

* * *

I think that a pregnancy center with an ultrasound scanner improves the chances of saving babies by a factor of at least two. For CPCs without ultrasound ability, there are "Going Medical" programs that are promoted by the national CPC associations. These programs are very complex, requiring long distance travel in order to train leaders and counselors and also requiring certification and oversight by hostile state bureaucracies. So-called "Going Medical" also requires full-time medical employees—a very expensive expansion. The idea behind these programs is that a CPC will hire a medical director and a sonographer, apply for a medical clinic permit from the state public health department, recruit a doctor to do physical examinations and read the ultrasound scans and otherwise turn the CPC into a full medical establishment with all the advantages and disadvantages and all the increased expenses. I think the first question for centers considering that option is "Where do we get the money for that kind of expansion?" And second, "Could we use that money otherwise to save babies?" And third, "Is 'Going Medical' the only way for CPCs to do ultrasounds?"

Problem Pregnancy has an ultrasound scanner. We are all volunteer and we did not use the "Going Medical" method. The least expensive method and least likely to bring hostile public bureaucracies down on a CPC is for the pregnancy center to become a doctor's branch office. To do that requires a very pro-life physician with full confidence in the CPC and a professional volunteer staff to do the scans. We do limited obstetric sonograms and specifically we never do any diagnoses. Clients sign release forms for many services at our center including sonograms.

The first ultrasound unit we bought was a demonstration model with only a few hours on it. We paid $25 thousand for it about ten years ago. In 2009 we were fortunate to be one of the first pregnancy centers to get into the Knights of Columbus National Ultrasound Program. The Massachusetts

Council and the Supreme Council (national) of the K of C split the cost and donated our new $30 thousand Biosound unit with much better resolution and thus a much better baby-save rate than our old tired unit. The scanner also has a Doppler (boom, boom, boom—the client hears the baby's heartbeat) and other added features. Biosound will not sell their scanners to abortion mills. That alone is a good reason to buy their equipment. Pro-lifer Jim Scheffler, (iit-jim@msn.com) is the Biosound distributor.

In the last year Problem Pregnancy has noted an unfortunate phenomenon among our ultrasound clients. Ten years ago the rate of abortion intent women changing their minds to life for their baby after seeing the ultrasound scan was 80 to 90 percent. The save rate today is still very good but the percentage is dropping. We don't know what to make of it because we have changed nothing. More babies die when that percentage goes down.

* * *

Attracting women college students (and other educated women) to your CPC is very important. In my city there are about 10 colleges and our center does not do a good job of getting the pregnant college women in. Serving those babies and their mothers is our responsibility too, as well the more financially needy women. National figures from CPC associations report that college women in general do not trust religious based organizations. Such women are bright and unfortunately many have often been negatively influenced previously by feminist propaganda.

Another factor is that they expect a professional office atmosphere. My advice is to segregate the baby boutique area of your center, so that it is not visible from the entrance or waiting room. Also different advertising and outreach is needed to reach these women. We advertise in every local college's annual directory, distributed to each student in September. In 2010 we ran a large ad in the Worcester College Student Survivor Guide. It is distributed to all incoming college students in September. It helps but we still need to do more. We also run weekly classifieds in the area's alternative newspaper.

A former director of Daybreak, a Boston area CPC once used this true anecdote about educated women clients in an appeal letter, "Carol was afraid. How could this happen to me? She looked in the Yellow Pages and found Daybreak. Carol was a young professional woman and she was sure she wanted an abortion. She came in for a pregnancy test over her lunch hour. She had questions about abortion procedures and their safety.

The counselor was able to connect with Carol closely enough to discuss risks, emotional scarring and the development of life inside her. Then she handed Carol a brochure full of great information that would further answer her questions. As Carol thumbed through the booklet, she seemed grateful for such accurate information . . . and then she turned to the last page. Across it was the name of the organization that printed the brochure. Among believers it was a reputable name. But because the word 'Christian' stood out so clearly to Carol, she tossed the brochure into the garbage, and walked out. In that instant, our opportunity to reach her was gone." The same feminist ideal of independence that approves of a successful career woman as a single parent, puts even more abortion pressure on the younger woman who has not yet achieved that success.

A Family Research Council market research study relating to CPC use is helpful to us in discovering the attitudes of more educated women. The study compares how pregnancy is perceived by the lower socioeconomic group vis a vis the higher socioeconomic group. The women's attitude of the poorer group, according to the study is, "The pregnancy is seen as yet another personal setback in an already hard life." And further from the study about the poorer women, "The sense of failure may be reinforced by the consequences, including the loss of ability to cope (socially, economically, personally) or the loss of the possibility of finding a decent man." Problem Pregnancy finds this type of client is seeking the resources necessary to help them survive and they like pro-life pregnancy centers.

On the other hand the study found the wealthier women to be goal-oriented and concerned about their careers. They are independent and fear becoming dependent upon others or being seen as a disappointment by family and peers. These women view CPCs as a health resource where they can find information on the various options, as well as clinical services. According to the study, CPCs, wanting to reach these women, need to demonstrate respectability, credibility and professionalism.

* * *

In my seventy one years some truths have been laboriously and painfully revealed. One of those important truths is that failure and success have certain characteristics when applied to human endeavors. By that I mean that successful people or successful business organizations or even successful crisis pregnancy centers exhibit recognizable hallmarks.

Usually the successful entity has had one person who has either pioneered it from its inception or taken it from a low point and turned it around. Not a committee. Not a board of directors. No – just one leader, her vision, her follow-through and her very hard work.

Another characteristic of success is now obvious to me but it took years of business experience before I noticed it – rigor. But how does rigor drive an entity to success? If you find a book that you think is great, it wasn't magic that produced it. Someone sat down and spent months or years writing that book, then rewrote it maybe ten times. Before he began writing, the author did long hours of research and spoke to many experts in the pertinent field. After he thought he was finished, the author probably gave it to editors who criticized it, revised it and used the delete button without mercy. Usually the author was unhappy (as I was) and reluctant but went along with those revisions. The final result of all that effort is the book that you like. That is rigor.

I have worked for industrial firms that were rigorous and very difficult to work for. They demanded almost super-human requirements of their employees. That type of company, if it also had tough goals up and down its whole company structure, would wipe out the competition every time. I've seen it. It's true. It's rigor.

It can be seen in sports when after a very rough four quarters and a tie score, the two football teams are beat-up and exhausted. But the rigorous team somehow finds the strength and fortitude to play the overtime with newfound energy and zeal and takes the win. It works with individuals also. When your eyes are blurring and you are worn out and it's eight o'clock at night and you been going since seven in the morning and you discover a math mistake in tomorrow's presentation, and it takes until midnight to get it right, you will most likely be successful in that effort. That is rigor.

And everyone wants to go to the surgeon who has a record of saving "doomed" cases. We have all heard of and some of us have been fortunate enough to have had such a doctor, using all his rigorously acquired knowledge and skill to operate with demanding discipline and ends up changing what had been a deadly prognosis.

On the other hand, just doing enough is the opposite of rigor. We all complain about slipshod restaurants, rude store clerks, incompetent government workers and arrogant politicians. It is so easy to fall into bad habits that we rationalize by thinking everyone else is doing it half-assed also. Good enough for government work isn't anywhere good enough.

So the pertinence for this book is that the abortionist has almost all the advantages in the competition for babies' lives. Those of us running crisis pregnancy centers in order to win at least some of the battles and save some of the endangered babies, must be rigorous in our efforts. By that I mean that we must set our offices up in the most advantageous manner that is possible within our means. We should train our counselors with the latest effective methods. We must instill in our volunteers the absolute need to save babies. We must research the enemy's methods of recruiting clients and operating his abortion business. We must know our competition so we can foil him where and when we can. We must go the extra mile. We must strain ourselves. Vigor should be added to rigor. We must be willing to be embarrassed and ridiculed. Sweat, blood and tears must be expended, yours not the babies. More babies will live if we are rigorous!

Board Members, Managers, Operations

To operate a CPC successfully, good business practices are necessary. A non-profit corporation is the best structure to operate a baby-saving office. There may be other structures that could be used, but in order to provide tax exemption for your supporters' donations, a 501(c) (3) corporation is necessary. Filing the right forms and recruiting the best board members and officers is a job for the leader. A certified public accountant (CPA) is another necessity since the IRS and other government officials need annual reports, showing the funds coming in and the expenses going out. Only CPAs have the credibility to produce audited reports accepted by all regulators. Also some intelligent donors want to know that your non-profit is legitimate and the proportion of operating expenses to income is below 25 percent. Most volunteer organizations will have no trouble with that proportion. I have never been able to find a pro-bono CPA.

Public Relations and Politics

Planned Parenthood is particularly good at getting undeserved good publicity. They work at it all the time. Most CPC operators are overwhelmed and undermanned (under-womanned?). We therefore get either no publicity or bad publicity. It is important, that we let the public know what we do. If we do the writing, it will be true and it will present our baby-saving, women-helping work in the best light. If the bad guys write it, we will get the shaft. Perception is reality in the media world. If a tree falls in the woods without TV cameras taping the various angles as it tumbles, it really did not fall. So don't count on scoffing the firewood for your fireplace.

How the local government officials perceive us, how other non-profits and the academy perceive us, and finally how the public perceives us, comes from newspaper, radio and TV media coverage. CPCs must be active in this regard. If you receive bad publicity, unwarranted or otherwise, respond to it quickly and strategically in writing or on TV, if possible. If your local abortionist receives warranted or unwarranted good publicity, think about a legitimate way to rebut it in writing. The rebuttal needs be true and believable or it won't be taken seriously.

Writing is a very important part of a pro-life leader's duties. Emailing has become very important in quick communications with allies. However, lucid, formal writing is also very important, such as letters to the editor, communications to donors and allies, opinion pieces, magazine articles, proposals for large donations, rebuttals to abortionists' good publicity, letters to elected officials about pertinent legislation and other public relations writing.

* * *

Most centers will be IRS tax exempt 501(c)(3) corporations and are not allowed to be involved in politics as an organization. Individual members of pregnancy centers are not so restricted. Planned Parenthood seems to ignore any such restrictions. It has its own tame legislature in Massachusetts. Everything it wants it receives, including a "loan" of millions of dollars with a probable no pay-back codicil to build its Worcester, Massachusetts abortion fortress. Other liberal states' legislatures are capons also, like California, New York, Connecticut, Maryland, Oregon, etc. Planned

Parenthood and NARAL are pretty good at gelding politicians.

Although we can't put political signs on our buildings, we as individuals can vote and we should. Be aware of the pro-life PACs and other allied organizations' political actions, so we know for whom to vote in or out of office.

I need a political favor. I have a request for the leaders of the pantywaist Congress and all the feminist controlled state legislatures. Would you please ask NARAL, pretty-please, if it would allow you to vote a change of date for the "National Day of Appreciation for Abortion Providers" now on March 10, to another day? It is my birthday, for Pete's sake!

Volunteer vs. Paid Management

There are definite advantages of having paid management run a CPC. Planned Parenthood has paid staff and they spend hours and plenty of money working to increase abortions and thwart pro-life efforts. Volunteers, on the other hand, have outside jobs, families and homes to run. Volunteers' time is generally much less than paid staff would provide. That deficit of time shows up especially in the lobbying efforts within local community groups and at local government meetings. Planned Parenthood seems to hammer us every time by associating with other more acceptable social agencies in joint projects and in getting favorable publicity.

I think of sales jobs that I have had and how I would get involved more and more in every facet of the job, the longer I worked at it. I would know my product cold and learn my competitors' weaknesses and strengths and tailor my sales efforts to those factors. I would learn shortcuts and tricks to be successful and to make my life easier. When we do something part-time, as a volunteer, we do not immerse ourselves. Since we are not at the abortion site every day, we miss things about the abortionist that could help our baby-saving. That is an unfortunate fact but even with that shortcoming, we still need to save babies as effectively as we are able.

Yet there are many offsetting benefits that a volunteer-run organization has. The dedication, the passion, the sense of duty of volunteers can't be bought with a paycheck. I still think that keeping the costs down at a volunteer-run pregnancy center both grows the new organization slowly and wins out in the comparison between paid staff and volunteer organizations. In the future the center could evolve into a larger outfit with paid staff.

In 1999, I went to a Heartbeat International CPC Conference near Baltimore. Problem Pregnancy has long been a member of Heartbeat, a national association of CPCs.

The conference went for four days. I picked the sessions that most interested me (fund raising, website development, etc.) and therefore spent only one day. There were other sessions aimed at tough counseling situations, adoption, and other things from which our counselors would have gained.

It was my first meeting with so many other centers (hundreds). I noticed that most of those CPCs had paid staff. In friendly conversations with other pregnancy center leaders, I was challenged that volunteer CPCs probably were less effective, than those with paid staff. I suppose I caused this challenge by my own bragging about Problem Pregnancy and our success at saving babies and helping women with our wonderful volunteer crew. Although inwardly I bristled, I decided to consider their criticism. I asked many questions of pregnancy center personnel and other leaders but remained puzzled as to which model was more effective.

So, when I got home I wrote a long letter to Dr. Peggy Hartshorn, President of Heartbeat International asking her to assess Problem Pregnancy in comparison with paid staff centers of similar size, budget, etc. I gave her our statistics for three years (number of pregnancy tests, women aided, turnarounds, budget, population, etc.). Dr. Hartshorn founded and is the chairwoman of a CPC, like ours in Columbus, OH, in addition to being the president of Heartbeat.

I spoke to her two weeks later. She said that she intended to write to me, but we hashed it out by phone instead. She said that it was hard to compare CPCs. One reason was that there are no standards on collecting statistics. For instance, our client statistics do not include our Hotline (call forwarders) telephone counseling and how many women were helped and how many baby-saves happened on the phone. Other pregnancy centers do count that type of counseling in their total number of women served.

She disagreed that paid staff type pregnancy centers are necessarily more effective. She said that the "passion" of the founding leadership of a volunteer center is one of the most important factors. She said that "the passion for saving babies" permeates such a CPC with its original founders, passing on to the newer counselors the same aggressive "do whatever we can to save the baby" attitude. She said that some pregnancy centers, without that passion and example, in some ways just go through the motions giving up too soon on the abortion minded women.

She said that our effectiveness shows up in the special statistical category of the large number of abortion minded women, who come to our center, thinking we are Planned Parenthood and how successful we are in turning them around. She thinks that our volunteers disprove any theory that paid staff is better. Her opinion, relayed to me, is that

Problem Pregnancy, as an all-volunteer center, is very effective, relative to other CPCs.

Real Estate

Finding the right real estate to open the CPC Plus will be formidable. I mentioned the New Women's Center in the "Naming Your CPC" section above. The organization began after a speech I made to the Pioneer Valley Massachusetts Citizens for Life in May of 2009. It was the 38th Annual Mothers' Day Dinner. I had been scouting the Springfield, Massachusetts streets for a CPC location around the Baystate Medical Center area, where Planned Parenthood is located. Baystate Medical is a hospital that has expanded into the Brightwood neighborhood to a formerly industrial, brown-fields urban area. That expansion has started a medical real estate boom. The area continues to grow with medical businesses. Older red brick industrial buildings are being demolished and new modern doctors' office buildings are going up.

Also that bonanza mentality, begun with the medical building expansion, has spilled over into new commercial building and substantial inflation of real estate prices has arrived. I was searching for a small, low rent, storefront near this booming area. I began this reconnaissance in 2005 soon after Planned Parenthood expanded into Western Massachusetts. This was just about the beginning of the real estate "gold rush." I was unsuccessful in finding a location close to the abortionist, mostly because all the small older buildings that had such proximity to the abortionist rental space had been razed to build the medical behemoths. Every few months I would drive and walk around the Brightwood neighborhood, looking for a proper site to no avail. The correct real estate is very important to the abortionists and to their pro-life competitors.

Without boring my reader completely with details, let me just say that in working on this project for years, I involved several groups of local people and discussed many possible permutations of a CPC but never got it going. So when I agreed to be the keynote speaker in Springfield at the largest pro-life dinner in Massachusetts, I accepted with an ulterior motive.

My speech was written to provoke an audience reaction. That hoped-for reaction was that local pro-lifers open a new CPC/Sidewalk Counseling Center very near Planned Parenthood in Springfield. In the speech, I explained the number of abortions done, the feeble response of Western Massachusetts pro-lifers to that carnage and the possible solution – a new pro-life center. The speech was about 20 minutes but I interrupted it about halfway through at the correct strategic point and asked volunteers to meet me after the speech in a particular corner of the hall. I was worried about angering the attendees, because my words were not flattering to local baby-saving efforts. After finishing the speech and listening to the surprising heavy applause, I looked over to the suggested meeting corner and voila! There was a large group of folks waiting for me. From that group has come the New Women's Center (NWC).

At this writing, NWC has already sent out the first of its four annual appeal letters and has been relatively successful. It has also has received its first large donor gift of $60 thousand. We were disappointed in our plans to raise $250 thousand+ to buy a building that would suit our needs. The building we had in mind, very close to Planned Parenthood, was sold to investors before we had our large gift. Presently we are negotiating for an office rental a little further away as an interim step. Maybe by the time this book is published, NWC will be saving babies at Calvary, please God.

Recently I spoke to a group of Catholics in Lawrence, Massachusetts, the cradle of American industry. While there I visited an independent abortionist's facility nearby. This doctor was strategically located at the end of a private road in the last building in a private, commercial office park. All pro-life presence was severely restricted. The few sign carrying, rosary bead thumbing protestors were frozen out and forced to stand more than a football field away, on the public sidewalk at the entrance to the office park. I've heard since that this doctor has quit that commercial building and moved to another commercial building in Haverhill, Massachusetts. A nearby rental is being contemplated for a new CPC by my friends, Fr. Benedict Hughes and John Cronin. Perhaps isolating his Lawrence abortion clinic from pro-lifers also isolated it from his potential clients. Sometimes abortionists are as error prone, as we are. We should take advantage when we can. I repeat that the correct real estate is very important to the abortionists and to their pro-life competitors.

In Hartford, Connecticut, I visited one of the area abortion mills, the Hartford Gynecological Center, just off Main Street on the south side of the city. In front of that abortion facility, like many other abortion facilities, there were a few faithful Christians, mostly Catholics, praying and trying to speak to the clients walking in to abort little innocent babies. Diagonally across a very busy and wide street, perhaps 50 yards away was a second floor, Catholic-operated pregnancy center. The woman, running that center is wonderful, holy and caring. However there are no inviting signs visible on her building aimed at abortion "clinic" clients across the street. The doorway and narrow entrance staircase and the general outside appearance of the CPC are uninviting and threadbare.

Yet next door to the abortion "clinic" was a commercial building with a for sale sign on it. I asked the volunteers, if anyone knew anything about the property, the price, etc. No one had any information. The location would be perfect in providing to a new pregnancy center, what I call Holy Spirit clients, those who come into the CPC by mistake. Also its first floor access would be much easier for sidewalk counselors to bring the ambivalent clients, rather than the traffic-filled trek across the street. Once again, I write that the correct real estate is very important to the abortionists and to their pro-life competitors.

There is a Planned Parenthood in Norwich, Connecticut just off the interstate. The neighboring buildings all house respectable medical offices. Abortionists like to appear legitimate by moving into buildings where doctors do real medicine. The medical building in which Planned Parenthood has its Norwich office also has such real doctors. Why would those doctors allow such a death camp in their midst? Why would the landlord rent to abortionists? There is a building for sale just across the narrow street from Planned Parenthood's parking lot. It is commercial and would be perfect for a CPC Plus. The correct real estate is very important da . da . . da. . da.

* * *

There are many sidewalk counseling efforts operating without a nearby CPC. Some are successful like Bill Cotter's Operation Rescue effort in Boston. Pro-life counselors in front of Planned Parenthood on Commonwealth Avenue, Boston and in front of Women's Health on Harvard Avenue in Brookline, Massachusetts are very effective. I think they could save more babies if they had an adjacent pregnancy center.

Emergency Mother Care (EMC) in New York City has sidewalk counselors at many abortion mills, not all proximate to a CPC. EMC is very creative. Chris Slattery, the director has a summer intern program, where college students are trained to do sidewalk counseling. He also uses fully equipped RVs with ultrasounds and professional counselors, parked in front of abortion facilities. One of those is the largest baby-killer in the east, Dr. Emily's in the Bronx. I've been inside those RVs and been in front of Dr. Emily's and other New York abortion mills with Slattery. He is the best baby-saver in the U.S.A.

I have seen pregnant women with shockingly noticeable bellies going into a late term abortion facility, Metropolitan Medical in Englewood, NJ. There were great Franciscan nuns in Englewood trying and sometimes succeeding in saving those viable infants, as little as two weeks before birth. The nuns had no nearby pregnancy center.

Project Defending Life is an Albuquerque, New Mexico group which has a multifold presence next to Planned Parenthood's abortion facility. This Catholic outfit has sidewalk counselors, pray-ers, a chapel fifty feet away and regular baby-saves.

There are two abortion mills in Providence, Rhode Island. Sidewalk counselors and prayers work hard at both sites and send the infrequent turnarounds to the two area pregnancy centers. My friend Dave O'Connell runs one, called the Mother of Life Center.

Advertising

Problem Pregnancy uses various media to let the target population know we are there to help. We have cut back our Yellow Page ads, but still use every contiguous yellow page book within 35 miles. Our ads under Abortion Alternatives are now much smaller, sometimes just a listing. We have saved money and it hasn't affected us adversely. We use the classifieds in alternative weeklies and the Spanish and African immigrant newspapers. We advertise under Pregnancy in all the college directories. Students constantly use those directories for take-out pizza or to find a dentist or a bookstore, etc. As I reported above, we ran a large ad in the Worcester College Student Survivor Guide in 2010. It is distributed to all incoming college students in September.

We have an internet site and we are tied into CPC networks, including Option Line, which heavily advertises its 800 number. We get local clients from that network, referred to our phone number. Our internet website is well done and we thank "A Woman's Concern," a well-run Boston CPC, for allowing us to use much of its content. We have a volunteer webmaster answering the emails from the website and forwarding the pertinent questions and information to the correct Problem Pregnancy person.

We are considering using the Worcester public bus system's inside transit ads but the bus company has had some difficulty with some of the wording in our ads. We want the word – abortion – to be in the ad. They don't. This kind of advertising is expensive. We have tried radio ads with not much luck. TV ads, until recently, have been out of our financial reach. We are reconsidering.

Signs

The pregnancy center's offer of services to pregnant women needs to be seen by the clients going into the abortion mill. Good, effective signs help to steal clients from the abortionist. Do not use churchy names, baby related words, the words "mother" or "life" or graphics of mothers and babies on the face of your main outdoor sign or any other sign. The wording on the sign should be neutral but women oriented. The colors should be woman attracting. My counselors tell me that purple is a good color for women.

Do not use the word "free." This is counter-intuitive and maybe a little controversial, but my experience says that today's more educated women think that there are government programs (read free) for almost everything. So, if your sign prominently states, that your services are free, those aware women, already warned by the abortionist to watch out for crazy Christians, might figure out that your center is not an abortion "clinic." We do not want that. In order to help those women, we need to talk to them. College women are alerted to Christian CPCs, learned from their so-called "Women Studies" courses.

"Pregnancy Services" in large letters, visible from a distance with the phone number, is ideal. The Holy Spirit will bring in the abortion intent women, if you give Him a little help with your location and a good sign. And don't forget to pray a lot also.

There are other signs involved in CPC work also. Outside almost every abortion facility, pro-life protesters will be carrying various signs; some homemade, some mass produced, some very graphic, some we don't like and some that are dog-eared and dirty from too much use. There are different schools of thought among pro-lifers about graphic signs showing bloody parts of aborted babies in real life colors. Some of us think, that those signs need to be seen because abortion is so hidden away that real bloody abortion results are never seen by the general public and need to be. Others think it causes our target clients to look away and move faster into the abortion "clinic" to get away from such signs. In other words, we might be losing our chances to talk to clients, because of those signs. If passersby do not like the graphic signs, tough luck on them. Notice that I only consider factors relating to saving babies. Later in the book, I will discuss sidewalk counseling in some depth. Most sidewalk counseling programs specifically ban signs of any kind nearby. Signs compete with the sidewalk counselors for the attention of the abortion intent woman.

Highway billboard signs are mostly aimed at the general public to sway opinion on abortion. The message and the graphics are targeted for a broader audience than our clients. Billboard signs are very expensive, if bought from the large billboard firms. "Billboards for Life" in Kentucky has a program to make your own at very low prices. Other kind of signs are "transit ads" that are seen inside and outside urban buses and trains that will catch just the right audience for either an abortion "clinic" or a CPC—that woman who can't afford a car and is pregnant and desperate.

There is a new kind of exciting sign now available called LED (Light Emitting Diode) signs. These LED signs are very visible in the daylight, can be seen at great distances. I think that in some abortion "clinic" situations, the external LED sign with changing legends would be very effective in passing pro-life information to abortion bound women. Currently the signs are used for business promotional displays As far as I know, they are not at abortion mills yet but maybe soon to appear at your local baby-killer.

I have an idea that probably won't work at our Worcester abortion site but maybe at some other site. Picture an LED sign attached to a computer keyboard, operated remotely by a dedicated pro-lifer watching the clients as they go into an abortion mill. The sign is in a location that is visible to those clients. A woman wearing a red hat is seen at a distance by the operator, as she walks toward the abortion "clinic." He types in the following that immediately shows up on the big electronic LED sign, "You in the red hat, please talk to that woman with the blond hair on the sidewalk. She can help you." I would love to see that tried out.

I have also been researching smaller one-man, LED signs to be carried like a front baby sling and powered with rechargeable battery power. Weight and size has precluded the idea so far but . . ? CPC operators need to be smart and creative and use correctly placed signs to save babies.

Shari Richard of Sound Wave Images and I are experimenting with Apple's IPad. Our sidewalk counselors are showing abortion clients Shari's excellent "Window on the Womb" color 3D ultrasound film footage on the easy-to-handle IPad with real babies moving around in utero. The idea is that those abortion minded women will see what is really growing inside them and change their minds from abortion. It is such a new project that we have no results to report yet. All CPCs need to keep up with technology.

Minimum Needs

There are minimum requirements to open a CPC; an office with parking, heating and air conditioning, a telephone; trained volunteers, a ladies room, office furniture, a private counseling room and a waiting area separate, so clients are not able to hear confidential client or office conversations. The costs of opening a pregnancy center will vary depending on the address in the city or town, where it will be located. There will be general monthly expenses that all centers must pay; rent, heat, electric, phone, postage, stationery, minimal advertising to start, maintenance, printed materials, miscellaneous, and do not forget Heartbeat International membership fees. Without an association membership, your pregnancy center does not get the Option Line benefit, which is internet and phone referrals from local clients.

One of our enemies, NARAL is mighty concerned about Option Line. This quote is from a January 2010 warning NARAL sent to its members, "One of the most potent tools that CPCs have at their disposal is the Option Line, a joint venture between Care Net and Heartbeat International that operates as a 24-hour call center and web tool that transfers or refers women to the nearest CPC. During its first month in operation, the Option Line received approximately 2,000 calls and since then has added instant messaging and email capabilities to its arsenal. The service currently receives about 16,000 calls a month."

Protestors, Pray-ers and The First Amendment

In the "Signs" section, I mentioned protestors carrying signs of their own. A pro-life leader will discover that our movement has many strong characters. The First Amendment of the U.S. Constitution applies to pro-lifers and its many characters also.

Most sidewalk counseling experts think that ancillary picketing, protesting and sign carrying by well meaning pro-life allies is counterproductive on the street in front of the abortionist. However the experts agree that nearby praying is very productive. Some signs are not helpful in saving babies. Picketing and protesting sends an anti-abortion message to public walkers and drivers going by but doesn't do much to save babies. I have been told by ordinary people, not involved in abortion, that they developed their opinion of pro-lifers from the protestors in front of the abortion facility. And those particular citizens' opinions weren't good. In spite of passersby's opinion, pro-lifers have the right to protest the killing of millions of unborn babies.

Somebody should tell those state legislators and governors of states with buffer zones that Christians are included in the First Amendment. Massachusetts has the most restrictive buffer zone in the U.S.A. No pro-lifer is allowed to stand or to speak to any client within 35 feet of an abortion "clinic" entrance. Anyone other than a pro-lifer is free to do so. The Alliance Defense Fund with the help of Problem Pregnancy and other Massachusetts pro-lifers is challenging that law in federal court.

A relatively new and growing phenomenon is "Forty Days of Life." It is a surging national organization whose ecumenical volunteers stand and pray outside abortion facilities twice a year for a 40 day period. Their participants are recruited from local churches. They are peaceful and prayerful and often are able to turn mothers from abortion, just by being at the "clinic" praying. Heartbeat International is teaming up with "Forty Days of Life" for the first time in 2010.

7.

Join An Existing CPC?

As I have previously written, my contention is that there must be a CPC Plus very near every abortion facility in America. If you want to volunteer, find such a correctly located CPC or help move an existing one next to an abortionist or start a new one next to an abortionist. There are pregnancy centers that are trying to relocate near an abortion facility but need help. Many others are happy in their suburban or small town locations. We should do a little research on the CPC before we volunteer. If the center is a 501(c)(3) organization, it will file IRS form 990 (annual report on its mission, its programs and its finances). It can be accessed online at Guidestar (www2.guidestar.org). You can evaluate a charity's spending on fundraising by comparing it with the charity's overall spending.

These small struggling local centers are often in need of one good volunteer that could make a big difference. Money is usually its biggest problem and an unpaid volunteer who can raise money is like a sunny day in January here in New England.

If a CPC is willing to move to a strategic location near an abortionist and you are able to raise the funds necessary to move it and operate it, you will be saving many babies by your volunteer actions.

Pregnancy Center Associations and Journals

I am going to be critical of pregnancy center journals and associations in this section with the following two caveats. There are many good things that the CPC associations do and many articles in the pregnancy center journals that are welcome and helpful. Unfortunately, this section will be the most controversial in the book among my own allies and colleagues, because I think pro-lifers can do better.

Too many pregnancy centers have taken a subordinate, almost flunky position vis a vis the national associations. Those CPCs act afraid and dependent, almost child-like.

We can save more babies! What we need is a written declaration of war by all of the pro-life pregnancy centers in America on all of the abortionists. Pro-lifers must set up a military-like campaign to defend the millions of American babies, slaughtered each year.

I notice that Minnesota (and Governor Tim Pawlenty) is having great success reducing abortions with a small public grant program ("Positive Alternatives") that gives practical aid to pregnant mothers mostly through CPCs. That is right in line with my idea of offering real (read expensive) aid.

Even President Barack Obama acknowledges the need for material help. In August 2010 he launched a program called the "Pregnancy Assistance Fund." We will wait to see if it will really helps to stop abortions. Other than Minnesota, I see no urgency to develop such a national plan by CPCs to defend those babies. Many pregnancy centers are located nowhere near the baby-killers. Some of those remote centers might process 100 women a year or less, probably none really endangered by abortion.

This state of war requires that every abortionist in the U.S.A. be plagued by a CPC, either next-door or very close (inches not miles). Centers should not be located in Elephant Foot, Idaho, hundreds of miles from the death camps. If a military tactician analyzed the total current pro-life effort as an answer to abortion in the U.S.A., he might quote Napoleon, "The logical end to defensive warfare is surrender." Where is the go-for-broke, frontline offense? Consider professional basketball games, as the opposing team gets the ball, the home team fans start screaming "De—fense, De—fense" What pro-lifers must do now is start screaming, "Off—ense, Of—fense." But first we need a functional team. That should be America's pregnancy centers.

But maybe the team is not ready. We seem to be curled up in the fetal position. Remember that a defensive curling up doesn't stop the brutal carving up of millions of our little brothers and sisters. There is a "scaredy cat" timidity that persists in many of today's CPCs. Quite a few centers have come out of churches and rely too much on ministers and lawyers for operating advice. Attorneys and a churchy attitude foster this timidity. Lawyers are hard-wired to be unable to let their clients do anything risky. Churches are afraid of losing congregants or financial support by being controversial. Churches are often unfamiliar with business tactics, public relations or military type strategies also. Pregnancy centers are not churches. They are the frontline of a culture war or they should be.

Thoughtful planned risk is what wins battles and saves babies. Pro-lifers should think and act like good bridge players. We should have a five-step approach to each hand of cards or any other endeavor: set your goal, make your plan, carefully identify what could go wrong, have contingency plans for each eventuality and finally implement the plan.

Non-violent and legitimate head-to-head competition with abortionists saves lives. I think that the combination of an aggressive CPC (new or relocated) very near an abortionist and a sidewalk-counseling group, also aggressive on the frontline, is the recipe for saving babies. This should be done legally, sometimes overriding the advice of lawyers and with the planned risk necessary to be successful. Our centers should be primarily concerned with saving babies from abortion and mothers from huge moral errors, and secondarily concerned with saving the souls of the pregnant mothers.

I hope this book gives hardheaded practical advice on how to intervene and bring clients, heading for abortions instead to our pro-life offices. In my experience the national pregnancy center associations offer office procedures, center policy and fundraising advice, etc. but give meager or no advice on frontline baby-saving tactics that would attract abortion minded women. We need to rein in the profligate killing of babies. Our centers need advice from experienced people about saving babies out on the street.

Problem Pregnancy receives various publications purporting to provide assistance to free pregnancy centers. In my opinion, most of the articles are repetitive, not very useful and the premises too often are wrong. For instance, an Evangelical national organization puts out a CPC journal. One of its 2005 articles, "The Urban Initiative" describes the need for pregnancy centers in inner cities and for an urban program to provide such centers. So far, so good. The article then explains why these new urban centers need to provide STD and HIV testing and other additional services. This advice does not focus on the main task of a pregnancy center – saving the baby!

I think that additional CPC services should not be offered, unless they enhance the possibility of saving the baby's life. Planned Parenthood already does STD tests. Doing what Planned Parenthood does *not* do, is what saves babies.

One thing Planned Parenthood and other abortionists do *not* do is provide *substantial*, free material aid to pregnant clients. Our pregnancy centers should add that as a service. Problem Pregnancy's mission statement is "We provide anything, the lack of which, is causing a pregnant mother to consider abortion." That often means expensive material and financial aid. That means offering money or paying for a client's practical needs, so she doesn't kill her baby. To some that might seem like bribing the woman not to have an abortion. Duh! I would not call it bribery. I would call it effective. Why don't we ask some saved teen-agers, are they pleased or unhappy that their mothers had taken "ransom money" to finish carrying them, rather than aborting them? How do you think that a grown up "fetus" would answer that? The result of paying for an abortion intent mother's needs is a live baby. How do you argue with a live baby girl?

Recently we paid about $45 hundred for a wedding. Not long ago we "ransomed" a little unborn girl from abortion by buying a washer and dryer for her mother. A few years ago, we saved a baby by paying for a brake job so our client could get to work. Just this week, as I finish this book in August

2010, I'm writing a $15 hundred check to an automobile dealer for a car. Why? Because a pregnant mother, after six visits to Problem Pregnancy with four ultrasound scans, was finally convinced not to kill her baby, by the offer of a car. These are just a few examples. For 28 years we've done such things. All of our services and expenses are related to saving a client's baby. Otherwise, we won't do them. Doing other things, not related to saving babies, takes time from the main focus and is counterproductive

Even worse, another CPC journal's article purported to be a primer on yellow page advertising for pregnancy centers. Almost everything written was wrong. Particularly wrong was the article's admonition as follows, "In the text of your display ad, never use a 'bait and switch' tactic to attract clients to your center. Be honest about what you are offering through your display ads. For example do not try to attract a client by appearing to offer abortions, then switch your story once she gets to your center." This advice was clearly not written by an experienced, urban sidewalk counselor and it is lethal to unborn babies.

I'm puzzled how this attitudinal misconception started. Perhaps years ago some, well meaning folks with no frontline abortion facility experience sat down and decided for their own centers, that counselors should answer every question a client might ask, "honestly and immediately." So far, so good. What if a client with an appointment for an abortion is in a pregnancy center by mistake, because the Holy Spirit brought her in? What if she is really antsy about religious agencies? What does your counselor do, when she hears the following question, "Do you do abortions here?" Most likely, if that question is answered "honestly and immediately," it would eliminate any chance to help that mother and save that baby from death. The woman would flee. The baby would die. What if you could put off answering that question temporarily and answer her question by asking your own questions and that could save the baby? Reality should hit your head as well as your heart. I think these journals are publishing the opposite of what is needed for our pregnancy centers. This kind of uninformed and mistaken advice has got into the CPC associations' literature, as if it is gospel. It isn't! It is wimpy and wrongheaded advice to our center operators who need courageous, savvy and baby-saving counsel.

If new centers take such advice and are so honest in their yellow page ads, that they admit in print, that no abortions are done at their office, then why would any abortion minded clients come to their office? It is ignorant and self-defeating advice! Of course, we should not be dishonest, but Christ expects us to be shrewd also. There is a sin of scrupulosity. That is when we so overdo our avoidance of sin, that we become obsessive and silly. St. Alphonsus Ligouri described scrupulosity as, "the groundless fear of sinning that arises from erroneous ideas." That yellow page advice fits his description of scrupulosity. That misinformation angers me because many new CPC staffers will take it as true, become sheep-like and then severely restrict their agencies' chances to save babies.

New pregnancy center people should be told, that because of past abortionists' pressure on Congress and yellow page publishers, all CPC ads are *already* restricted to the *Abortion Alternatives* category by those publishers. The blame for that yellow page restriction should be laid exclusively on Senator Ron Wyden of Oregon, who carried the abortionists' water, regarding that legislation.

Problem Pregnancy's yellow page ads are purposely ambiguous. Most of our clients think we do abortions, although we never state so in our ads' text. Also in our office, when that direct question is asked and after we have tried to steer the conversation away without success, then we will tell the client that we do not commit abortions. We never volunteer that information. That would be like giving cyanide to our babies. We think of them as our babies. We save over 200 of them every year.

We are successful because of our aggressive attitude that we will do whatever (morally and legally) we must to save those endangered babies. We do sidewalk counseling, parking lot counseling and lots of praying outside the abortionist's office. We have a chapel with the Holy Eucharist resident with much prayer and adoration going on. We use fixed signs aimed at women across the street going in to kill their babies. We have an unconstitutional 35-foot buffer zone with which to contend. Planned Parenthood has sued us many times, yet we continue to save babies, despite all of the enemies' legal, political, legislative and other tactics.

In the same journal another article suggests that pregnancy centers ask Walmart or Pampers to help pay for their yellow page ad by adding the company trademarks in the ad. That is also deadly to babies for the same reason. In order to get abortion minded women into a CPC, we must provide no evidence to potential clients, that we are pro-life. The abortion intent woman (our target population) will run to the nearest abortionist, if she sniffs pro-life or Christian motives. Mentioning Pampers (a baby product) is a no-no. This target group of women will never call our office, if they see baby related items in our ads.

In our center's waiting room, we must constantly remove cutesy-poo baby clothing, dolls, holy pictures, church magazines, religious tracts, newspaper clippings, etc., all left by well-meaning volunteers. That kind of stuff is evidence to the abortion-intent women in our office by mistake that we are pro-life. That unborn baby's mother will run across the street to Planned Parenthood and kill her baby if she sees such paraphernalia. Therefore the article is counter-productive to the mission of pregnancy centers – saving babies.

I found another example of this timorousness coming from a pro-life legal advisory organization to pregnancy centers in a 2010 article called, "Fake Clients." The piece warns CPCs to train our receptionists and counselors to respond "honestly and factually" to every inquiry. The article states, "If the telephone caller asks if you do abortions, clearly answer that you do not perform or refer for abortions." Why would pregnancy centers tell abortion-minded women to go elsewhere? To an abortion mill? That's what that legal advisory outfit recommends. Don't pay any attention to that dopey advice. I write about how to handle fake clients further on in the book.

Our CPC has been regularly smeared in the media and evicted once, because of Planned Parenthood's pressure on our landlord. But we've become very savvy about the opposition. For example, a few years ago we bought the building that we had been renting adjacent to the abortionist so we could never be evicted again. We, battle-scarred veterans understand that we are located at Calvary and that real babies' lives are the *price* of losing any of the one-on-one battles with our abortion intent clients. We take that responsibility very seriously. *If we lose a battle, the counselor doesn't die. I don't die. The CPC journal editor doesn't die. The legal advisor doesn't die but a real little boy or girl dies, painfully.* Those advising journals and advisories need to very careful, that their advice does not cause babies' deaths.

Some pregnancy centers should consider getting out of the CPC business and starting a church. I mean those centers that operate to that misconceived and fearful standard rather than trying to stop the massive killing of babies. There should be evidence that your center is effective. Abortionists and their allies should be calling the police on your center or writing nasty letters to the editor or painting graffiti on your building or suing you. That's your *report card.*

Our history suggests the following hypothesis: the effectiveness of your pregnancy center should be measured by how much trouble is visited upon your center by Planned Parenthood, NARAL or other abortionists, its allies and its legal machine. The more grief and trouble you are getting, the better you must be doing in saving babies. If your CPC is not getting a bad time from abortionists and our other enemies, then you are not very effective in saving babies. You need to stick your finger in the abortionist's eye, figuratively speaking. They are killing babies! We should be throwing chairs and stomping on the floor, metaphorically, that is. Save babies and take business away from them! Write nasty letters about them! Sue them! We should not be their punching bag. Show some bare knuckles and some spine. The more difficulty you get, the better you are doing as a baby-saving center. Our center gets an A on our *report card.* How about yours?

If the CPC national associations want to aid pregnancy centers, show them how to move next door to abortion facilities or help pro-lifers learn how to sidewalk counsel at the death camps. Teach them to save babies on the frontline. A recent example—Problem Pregnancy saved four babies from Planned Parenthood during the holiday week of July 4, 2010. God is powerful and helps those who are saving babies. If the effort to move next door to abortionists seems to be too difficult, pray, have faith in Jesus Christ and listen to Mother Teresa's comment on lack of funds, "God has plenty of money."

8.

"To achieve great things, we must live as though we were never going to die" Marquis de Vauvenargues

Starting and Operating a Combination Frontline Center

I have coined a phrase for the combination CPC and sidewalk counseling effort. I call it CPC Plus. I write this, as if a new CPC Plus was needed next to an abortion mill in an American city and I was asked for advice. In fact, that is exactly what is happening in Springfield, Massachusetts, as I mentioned before. I have been involved with the "planting" of many new and relocated pregnancy resource centers. I will tell you how one such center began.

In Chapter 6 under Real Estate, I mentioned the New Women's Center, the start-up in Springfield, Massachusetts. Below is more on that CPC. For five years I have been trying to start a CPC Plus in Springfield, next to Planned Parenthood's abortion mill. Over 3 thousand babies are destroyed there with no nearby CPC to which to bring ambivalent clients. There are a few heroic sidewalk counselors and pray-ers, freezing and sweltering outside the "clinic," depending on the season, trying to save babies. Since beginning in 2009, the New Women's Center Inc. (NWC) has made great progress in organizing a non-profit corporation, getting its federal tax exemption, searching for a location and beginning to raise funds to rent or buy that building. The staff will be all volunteer and the counseling training has begun. The volunteers understand that a Sidewalk Counseling component is necessary to save up to ten percent of the 3 thousand babies killed. Although there hasn't been a grand opening, I think the NWC is a good model to use as an example of starting from scratch. More information on this start-up is interspersed in the sections below.

How Do We Begin to Sidewalk Counsel?

I am fortunate to have taken two different Sidewalk Counseling training sessions directly from the two masters of the subject; Ann Scheidler of the Pro-Life Action League, Chicago and Monsignor (Msgr.) Philip Reilly of the Helpers of God's Precious Infants of Brooklyn. I have also had 28 years of on-the-job-training. I confess that I'm not very good at turning young women away from abortion. Almost any woman is better at it than I am. Much of the following comes from written material from Ann Scheidler and the Chicago method. There is another section in this book after this one on Msgr. Philip Reilly, the Helpers method and some Karen Black ideas. I've used material from these masters and some from my own experience. There are other sidewalk counseling training programs also.

Sidewalk counseling takes place in front of an abortion facility. It is a method of saving babies by talking to their mothers and to those arriving with the mothers. It is the single most valuable activity that a pro-life person can engage in. When we counsel in front of an abortion clinic, we are coming between the woman and the abortion doctor; between the baby who is scheduled to be chopped up and the abortionist who would do the chopping if we are unsuccessful in stopping it.

Counseling goes to the very heart of the abortion problem. The problem of abortion is that it kills babies. They are killed mostly in dedicated abortion facilities. Some abortionists also operate as doctor's offices and some abortions are committed in hospitals. Frontline pro-lifers intercede for the baby's life, wherever the killing happens. As you know by now, the aim of this book is to get more people out on the streets to stand between the killers and the victims.

There are many effective ways to do sidewalk counseling. Whatever the individual counselor's specific tradecraft, she has to know something about human nature and must be able to understand the crisis a pregnant woman is facing. The counselor should understand the mother's reasons for making this unnatural decision to rid herself of her baby by abortion. We know that the worst solution for her is to kill an innocent human being and that is what a woman chooses in having an abortion. What drives her to do that? We need to know that. Is it such a difficult decision to make, that once it is made, there is no way to turn back? That is not true. Women *can* be turned back. Thousands of people are alive today because a sidewalk counselor or a crisis pregnancy counselor helped their mothers to choose life. In Chicago, in one thirty-day period, half a dozen sidewalk counselors at only a few "clinics" were able to stop ninety women from having abortions. I dream that sidewalk counselors will be present at all abortion "clinics" in the U.S.A. during all open hours.

If you were driving by a school and saw a man struggling with a group of children, trying to snatch a little boy, what would you do? Would you write a letter to the editor? Would you tell your neighbors about it at a weekend barbeque? Would you write to your congress-man? Would you demand better police protection in your neighborhood? No! You would stop your car, immediately start hollering and run over try to directly stop the abduction and save the boy. If this culprit ran into a building with the boy, you would go into that building. You would go where the child is and try to save him.

That is what sidewalk counselors do when they go to an abortion clinic. The unborn baby is as alive and as human as that schoolboy struggling with a kidnapper. We need to put ourselves between the child and the abortionist. Before we do that, however, we must develop the knowledge and the skill, to actually have a chance to save the child. We have to save the child outside the "clinic" through our words, our actions, the correct attitude and lots of prayer. I can't think of any action at an abortuary, that is more direct and is also legal.

There are people at abortion clinics, whose only job is to pray for the mothers, the babies, the counselors and that the abortion staff will repent and stop the horror. That prayer is very effective. It positively affects the people going by and the people going in the abortionists. Prayer has it own special power and it is always essential. Some of us pro-lifers have a special calling and the skill to reach out and talk to the pregnant woman, the boyfriend, the parent, or friend who is accompanying the young woman. Frequently a woman, accompanying the abortion client, has had an abortion herself and is very defensive about it. Increasingly we find that the pregnant woman, herself, has had a previous abortion. These facts often make the job more difficult for us.

Time is crucial as a woman approaches the abortion clinic. The counselor should quickly and politely ask the woman, if she wants to talk. If the woman says no, that should *not* be the end. A good salesman would say to himself, that *no* is "the beginning of the sale." I think that counselors should develop that same dogged attitude. Try to win the woman over again in other ways, like offering her literature or providing her with life-saving information. The experts recognize that by the time a woman arrives at the abortion facility, she has already mentally aborted her baby. She often sees herself in an impossible situation.

The Chicago experts developed an approach, grounded in the realization, that women at an abortion clinic are more concerned about their own health and safety, than they are with their babies. We need to present to the woman how dangerous the abortion procedure is to her. That there are physical and psychological consequences to her following an abortion. To further emphasize the dangers, research needs to done on malpractice lawsuits that may have been filed against the abortion doctors and the "clinics" where they work. Summaries of those collected legal complaints need to be distributed to clients approaching the clinic and to those accompanying her, who should be concerned for her safety.

Usually the records are available at the District or Superior Courts and are public records. There are often records of malpractice lawsuits for many injuries from abortion procedures: perforated uterus, excessive bleeding, failure to diagnose an ectopic pregnancy, puncturing an artery, and even death.

The Chicago Method people use these records as their basis. The sidewalk counselor or others should regularly check the court records to uncover recently filed lawsuits. The researcher should read the complaint and summarize the allegations into a short paragraph. Compile the summaries into a list and distribute it to the abortion facility's potential clients, as they approach the "clinic." Include the file case number in your summary so that anyone, wishing to check up on the veracity of the claim, can easily find the record.

With this lawsuit information, the sidewalk counselor can approach a pregnant woman and perhaps speak to her like this, "Excuse me. Do you have an appointment at this clinic? Do you know about the medical malpractice lawsuits against this place?" The sidewalk counselor would then hand the woman and her companion the compiled list of legal actions against that particular abortion clinic, emphasizing that women have sued the clinic and the doctor for injuries that they have suffered. Any deaths at the facility should be highlighted. Keep an eye out for inevitable bad publicity about the abortionist or the "clinic." Make photocopies of any such newspaper articles to hand out at the clinic.

Regularly there are complications during abortion procedures, resulting in ambulances at the clinic. Pro-lifers should photograph such events. It's also advisable to film any incident of harassment at the clinic. An eight by ten copy of a picture of attendants taking a woman from the clinic and loading her into the ambulance can be shocking to an abortion intent woman.

A sidewalk counselor should tell the client after giving her the malpractice lawsuit list that she can recommend a safe pregnancy center close by (we hope), where the client can get a free pregnancy test and speak to a professional counselor. Assure her that the center works with doctors, who have clean records and have not been sued.

Once the woman or her companion appears willing to talk with the sidewalk counselor, the subject of the baby can be discussed. We have discovered that often a young woman doesn't realize that she is carrying a well developed life inside her at her stage of pregnancy. The abortionist's staff has probably told her that her baby is only tissue. They probably have lied to her to make her agree to the abortion. Abortionists need to do abortions to stay in business. They have nothing to gain by revealing to the client how magnificent her unborn baby actually is. Why lose a customer?

The sidewalk counselor should have literature with photos of the unborn baby at various stages of development with a description of the baby's capabilities. Sometimes a woman will have told herself, that if God doesn't want her to have this abortion, He will put someone in her way. There are times when all it takes to save a baby, is for you to be there with the facts of fetal development and the facts about abortion and be a willing to approach the abortion bound woman with those facts.

The woman should be encouraged to talk about her situation in order to find out the reasons, why she thinks abortion will solve her problem. Sometimes the sidewalk counselor can appeal to the boyfriend or husband to protect the woman and his baby. Sometimes the companion who has come with the woman can be the sidewalk counselor's ally in the effort to turn her from the abortion clinic.

My plan requires that a pregnancy resource center (CPC) be nearby. The waffling woman should be immediately taken to the center by the sidewalk counselor. The center will offer a free pregnancy test to confirm the pregnancy. The sidewalk counselor should encourage the woman to get this confirming test at this objective center. CPCs receive no money no matter which decision (life or death) the mother makes.

The kind of pregnancy center I recommend will help the woman with ancillary problems that often are the real cause of her seeking an abortion. The sidewalk counselor needs to know, what are the likely things that the center could do for her client. For example, the sidewalk counselor should not promise her that the pregnancy center would find a job for her. But at my center you could tell her that our center can provide her with vocational information, medical aid, legal help, immigration help, financial aid, housing help, maternity clothes, a baby crib, a car seat and other such amenities. Ideally, CPC will have a neutral-sounding name like "Pregnancy Services Center."

If the woman asks whether the pregnancy center offers abortions, be noncommittal by saying, "First they will do a pregnancy test to make sure you really are pregnant. Then they will do an abortion consultation and discuss your reasons for considering abortion and the risks involved. They will look at all your options. Perhaps they will do an ultrasound first to see how far along you are."

Many pregnancy resource centers have on-site ultrasound available. Others refer their clients to a nearby allied clinic, where an ultrasound could be done. The facts are that if an abortion-intent woman sees her baby on ultrasound, she is far less likely to opt for an abortion.

Sometimes the abortion bound woman will not be willing to go to the CPC but is willing to continue talking. Sitting in a car or just walking away from the abortionist is a good idea. If there is a coffee shop nearby, invite her to go there with you and talk about her situation.

Once the sidewalk counselor has established a relationship with the pregnant woman, they may exchange phone numbers. The mere fact that the counselor has shown a willingness to be available and supportive may be enough to help the woman decide to choose life for her baby.

Without real compassion for the pregnant mothers, the sidewalk counselor will not be successful in saving babies. By putting herself in the woman's shoes and listening carefully often the counselor will help the pregnant woman find her solution simply by talking out her concerns. Withholding judgment is very important in these initial conversations with the pregnant mother.

The sidewalk counselor is the antidote to the abortion facility staff that are paid to convince the woman to abort her child. The pro-life counselor should be a person with a strong sense of morality and an understanding of the long-term effects of a decision to have an abortion. Abortion stops a life that would eventually involve thousands of other lives. Ending a pregnancy ends generations.

Whenever a sidewalk counselor helps a woman reject abortion, she and all pro-lifers involved celebrate a "save." Sometimes the counselor might think she has lost and the baby will be killed. She might never know of the impact on a woman, she had, even after the client walks into the "clinic." Abortion clinic workers report that pregnant mothers often after spending hours in an abortion facility end up changing their minds, because of the influence of a sidewalk counselor. The counselor may also persuade those accompanying the pregnant woman. Good things often happen when a sidewalk counselor is able to talk to an abortion-intent woman.

Using versions of the Chicago Method, the Helpers of God's Precious Infant's method or other programs, American sidewalk counselors have saved thousands of babies from abortion by turning their mothers away from abortion clinics. We need to substantially increase the number of trained personnel in front of abortion facilities. There are different situations at "clinics" depending on the state or local laws. Harassment and lack of access for sidewalk counselors wanting to speak to abortion clients makes some "clinic" situations difficult. Buffer zones or bubble zones, police harassment and building layout or structural restrictions are a few of those difficulties. But we must overcome those disadvantages.

Prospective sidewalk counselors should know that once a woman has made the decision to go to an abortion clinic, her principal concern becomes her own health and safety, emotional and physical. Recognizing this reality, counselors seek to point out to the woman the many dangers of abortion to her and that it is always a bad decision.

Encountering a potential client turnaround as far away from the clinic door as possible is very important. When you see a client approaching walk quickly to meet her since she might rush past you, if she gets close to the "clinic." The abortionist's staff probably has told the client, when she made her appointment, that she should ignore anyone who tries to talk to her on her way in. She might be on-guard to ignore the counselor. If the woman refuses to stop and talk with you, try to get the point across that the clinic has many lawsuits against it and that you are simply warning women of the dangers they face. Your warning may be enough to make her consider the consequences of her choice, even though she may go into the clinic.

The pregnant woman's companion is often a key to saving the baby. She may go in and out of the abortion clinic several times while the client is inside. The atmosphere inside an abortion facility is stressful. No one wants to remain inside an abortion "clinic" very long. You will see them outside having coffee or smoking. The sidewalk counselor may be able to appeal to the boyfriend, the mother or father, or another companion, to hand pro-life information to the client. Working on the companion to understand the risks of abortion and getting him or her to take responsibility for the mother's safety, you may develop an ally to help save the baby's life. During your conversations with the companion show him or her the photographs of the unborn baby in the womb and after having an abortion. At this point in the process it is time to pull out all the stops. Emphasize the danger of abortion to the woman and describe the pain and death of the baby. Since you cannot go into the clinic, but the companion can, urge him or her to take on the mission of saving both mother and baby from the horror of abortion.

A new documentary (2009) called "12th and Delaware" is available that shows the raw life and death drama of Pregnancy Care Center, a Catholic CPC on one corner and

Woman's World, an abortion facility on the other corner of 12th and Delaware Streets in Fort Pierce, Florida.

Coincidentally, in 2008 Rachel Grady of Loki Films, the co-director of "12th and Delaware", and I were very close to having Worcester's Problem Pregnancy and Planned Parenthood be the antagonists of her film. We declined after much thought, with Kathy Lake, our nurse and my son, Rod Jr., himself a documentary filmmaker, both advising not to take the chance that the film would be a hatchet job. Although some CPCs think the movie is biased, I am surprised how relatively fair it is. I recommend the film to anyone thinking of taking up my challenge to open such a pro-life center. You will see how difficult, exhilarating and heartbreaking this God inspired work is.

Restricting the number of pro-life contacts, with which an abortion intent woman communicates, is important. Two sidewalk counselors working each clinic entrance is ideal. More than two counselors may be intimidating to the woman who is probably already nervous. No one other than trained sidewalk counselors should speak to the client. Pray-ers should pray only. Other pro-lifers should not be near the entrance and should be quiet. It is counterproductive, if the client hears loud yelling and seeming chaos from the people outside the "clinic." She will flee into the abortionist's office and the baby will be lost. It is often effective for one counselor to speak to the woman while the other speaks with her companion. This accomplishes two goals. You have a double opportunity to get the important information into the heads and hands of the couple on the way to the abortion, and you separate them from each other, so that if one of them is hesitant about the abortion, you can capitalize on that fact.

Sometimes the woman or her companion will claim that the abortion is necessary for health reasons. The counselor should respond that the worst place for someone with serious health concerns is an abortion clinic. The nearby CPC can hook them up with a doctor trained to handle high-risk pregnancies to make sure that she is well cared for. Mostly the "health" excuse is phony but it gives the opportunity to discuss an alternative to abortion.

The objective of the sidewalk counselor is to get the abortion intent client away from the abortion clinic as fast as possible. Spending too much time with one client may cause the counselor to miss other potential turnarounds. If you succeed in talking the woman out of the abortion, at least for the moment, get her to the pregnancy center as soon as possible. The counselor should accompany her and introduce her to the receptionist or the counselor and then leave the client in their hands. The sidewalk counselor can give her phone number to the client if it will help. Then return to your post on the sidewalk.

If the sidewalk counselor does her job correctly, very rarely will she get a hostile response from abortion bound clients, because the pro-life effort is low-key and it focuses on the health and safety of the pregnant woman. It leaves the door open for future communication with those who go in and later come out because they have second thoughts.

* * *

"The method of the Helpers of God's Precious Infants" is another regimen of sidewalk counseling. It uses Roman Catholic sacramentals and the Mass, along with its baby-saving efforts. In 1979, Monsignor Philip J. Reilly of Brooklyn, New York founded the Helpers. This group encourages pro-life people to pray and sidewalk counsel outside of abortion facilities. In spite of health problems, Msgr. Reilly has traveled the world, teaching the Helpers' method and now has Helpers' chapters in every major city in the United States and in many other countries.

Below I have described the Helpers method, using Reilly's literature. The Helpers Method consists of three interdependent activities: sidewalk counseling, intense prayer at the abortion clinic and remote spiritual supporters. According to the monsignor, prayer is the Helpers' most important activity. Praying outside an abortion "clinic" demonstrates publicly that all life is sacred. Freezing in the winter and sweltering in the summer at the abortion site unites Helpers with the suffering of the condemned unborn babies. Prayers by Helpers are in reparation for the injustice against those innocent babies. The Helpers see themselves as the Blessed Mother, St. John and St. Mary Magdalene, praying at the foot of the Cross. The prayers, from those Helpers may be the only show of human love those unborn babies will ever have in their short lives. The Helpers also pray for the conversion of the abortion-intent mother and father. According to the Helpers, there are many reports that women have changed their minds because of people praying for them at an abortion facility. Helpers also pray for the conversion of the abortionists and their staff. Sidewalk counselors and other pro-lifers need prayer also and the Helpers fill that need also.

The Helpers' method is a regular occurrence outside the target abortion facility but it also includes special occasion Prayer Vigils with a bishop or priest to celebrate Mass at a church near an abortion clinic. The Helpers coordinator must secure a parade permit from the police department for a procession from the church to the abortion clinic. The bishop would celebrate the Mass and lead the processing congregation in prayer over to the abortion "clinic." The congregation is asked to remain silent, except for the prayers led by the bishop and other designated leaders. The prayer group recites the twenty decades of the Rosary with hymns between each, as they walk to the clinic, where they will spend an hour of prayer. The only posters or graphics included in the procession are pictures of the Divine Mercy or Our Lady of Guadalupe.

In fact, no graphic abortion pictures and posters with written messages are allowed by the Helpers, either during regular sidewalk counseling or during the Prayer Vigil. Another of the Helpers' rules is that designated sidewalk counselors *only* are in contact with "clinic" clients. No socializing or visiting during prayer time is the Helpers' rule since the purpose is to manifest the power of God and the presence of the Holy Spirit. Prayer groups do not hold signs or call out to clients. While the prayer group is engaged in prayer, pairs of sidewalk counselors approach the pregnant mother and her companions. The Helpers' counselor offers a Rosary to the woman and to any companions, along with a leaflet about praying the Rosary. She might say, "No one really wants to be at an abortion clinic and praying the Rosary is a good way to ensure that you will not be back at an abortion "clinic" again." Otherwise, the sidewalk counselors use similar rules to the Chicago Method.

Those who attend the Mass, but are unable to join the procession, are invited to remain in the church in prayer, during the hour the others spend in front of the abortion facility. A Helpers' Prayer Vigil requires careful planning. Posters and invitations should be sent to all the parishes in the area. The coordinator should contact the various parish Respect Life directors for assistance in promoting the Vigil. Hymn sheets need to be prepared. Future sidewalk counselors and prayer group members need to be recruited via the Helpers' Prayer Vigil. Sign-up cards should be distributed at the Prayer Vigil Mass for this purpose.

At the abortion site, Helpers use a prayer book compiled by Msgr. Reilly and dedicated to the Precious Blood of Jesus. The book is divided into three hours of litanies, Scripture readings, Stations of the Cross and the Rosary. The prayers are taken from traditional Catholic sources, as well as the Bible. so that Catholics and non-Catholics may pray together, according to Helpers' literature. Groups may pray for three hours or less at the abortion clinic. Some spend an hour, once a week or once a month. Most prayer groups meet on Saturdays because more people are available but any day is a good day to pray.

A Helper never prays alone. Without a witness, there is the risk of being falsely accused of wrongdoing by abortion clinic staff. Abortionists are notorious for falsely accusing pro-lifers of assault, etc. to rid their facility of opponents. There should always be at least two praying together.

Helpers also recruit others who can't be at the clinic to pray, such as cloistered nuns and mothers at home with young children. These homebound supporters join their prayers with those of the sidewalk counselors and the abortion site prayer groups, according to the Helpers' literature.

The Helpers' suggestions regarding police communication should apply to all sidewalk-counseling programs. The Helpers state that it is a good idea to meet with your organization's lawyer and the police commander responsible for the abortion location where the sidewalk counselors and pray-ers will be. The police will then know who your group is, when and where it will be gathering and what it will be doing. Helpers emphasize that its group respects the law and will peacefully exercise their right to pray.

A positive rapport with the police is important. The abortion mill staff may call the police and report your activities as unlawful. Of course, they want to get rid of any pro-life presence. If police have already been contacted and apprised of what will happen, then the police will know that such activities are peaceful and lawful. Police must respond if the abortion clinic makes a complaint. There should be one designated Helpers' person to communicate with the police. Let the officer know that you have met with the precinct commander. It would be helpful to get the commander's business card in advance to show to the beat cop, if necessary. Assure the officer that you respect his authority and ask him to protect your First Amendment rights.

Helpers pray on public property at a spot that will not be distracting to the sidewalk counselors. Pray softly so as not to distract a sidewalk counselor trying to speak to an abortion bound woman. Do not block the sidewalk. The First Amendment of the Constitution protects public prayer. We thank the Helpers' and Pro-Life Action League. See contact information.[*]

* * *

Karen Black of Women4Women (Duluth, GA) has a website that asks a very pertinent question of sidewalk counselors – "Why am I out here in front of this abortion clinic?" She says it's not a fun place there on the sidewalk.

---

[*] Helpers of God's Precious Infants
5300 Fort Hamilton Pkwy
Brooklyn, New York 11219
718-853-2789 http://helpersbrooklymw.org

Pro-Life Action League
6160 N. Cicero Ave.
Chicago, Illinois 60646 773-777-2900 wVlw.prolifeaction.org

Karen Black, WOMEN 4 WOMEN

She tells of someone asking her to "give a pep rally" to sidewalk counselors. She declined and said, "It's not fun. It can be gut-wrenching. And your feet hurt, your back hurts, and you get friendly little hand signals all day. But it's not supposed to be fun. It may be the hardest thing you'll ever do. But it's also the most rewarding thing. When you've got that beautiful little baby in your arms and you know . . . . even if getting that mom to choose life for that child may have been stressful to you—it was worth every single moment of it." Karen Black says that we are out there because we want to save babies. That's a good reason. And she says, we are out there because we are obeying God when He says, "Don't stand back and let the innocent die" That also is a good reason.

Celebrity Sidewalk Counselors

During the writing of this book, I attended a May 2010 meeting of Problem Pregnancy counselors. The meeting's purpose was that we better use "Bella," the 2007 #1 top rated movie to help abortion intent women change their minds towards life for their babies. "Bella Hero" is a non-profit organization founded by the makers of "Bella" to help CPCs show the pro-life case to abortion minded pregnant mothers. Eduardo Verastigui, the heartthrob actor and star of Mel Gibson's "The Passion of Christ," is the leading man in this abortion related film. The movie is very clear that life for the unborn baby is the right choice among pregnancy options for the leading lady who becomes pregnant in the film. "Bella Hero" donates the DVDs to centers and we give them free to our clients, who take them home to watch. The film subtly makes our pro-life case to the ambivalent clients in the comfort of their own homes.

At that meeting with the "Bella Hero" representative I discovered something that later triggered an idea from my wife, Jean. We were told that Eduardo Verastigui is himself a sidewalk counselor whenever he gets a chance. Jean's half-humorous, half-serious idea was that we should recruit "Celebrity Sidewalk Counselors" to save babies at abortion mills. I've taken it one better. How about a reality TV show, "Baby-Saving with The Stars," shot in front of Planned Parenthood in Worcester with President George W. Bush, Nick Cannon, the pro-life rapper, Governor Sarah Palin, opera singer Andrea Boccelli and actors Patricia Heaton and Jon Voight on the busy, traffic filled, city street corner, competing to see who is the best at sidewalk counseling? Eduardo and I would be judges for that show. A score of one baby saved earns a Mother Teresa trophy. Of course, we would strive to award six trophies. Speechifying, singing and dancing would be optional!

In my almost thirty years outside abortion facilities, I've developed opinions on many things related to saving babies at Calvary. For instance, I think nuns in habits are the best baby-savers on the abortion front-line. We in Worcester pray for a new order of sisters, dedicated to sidewalk counseling and we have an empty convent waiting. The gentle but tough-minded maternal laywoman is the next best. In my opinion, women are much better at getting abortion intent clients to talk to them, as they go into an abortionist. These confused, distraught and often desperate pregnant mothers are focused on one thing – getting that abortion. Attracting their attention to discuss alternatives is very difficult. Priests or ministers with clerical collars and garb are the next best. Clients seem to be thinking clergy or nuns in habits would be sympathetic and will often come over to these counselors voluntarily. These clients are often upset at a particular man (for instance, the father of the baby who has put the client into this desperate situation) and at men in general. Men are the least successful in trying to get the clients' attention and therefore in saving babies. However, there are exceptional people, men and women, who continually save babies on the frontline.

To illustrate the fact that men are not the best sidewalk counselors, let me tell a real life story. This happened a few years ago at the Problem Pregnancy office. It was early on a Thursday morning. Barbara (pseudonym) was inside at the reception desk. Peggy (pseudonym) was outside doing sidewalk counseling. I'm over 6 feet tall and weigh over 200 lbs. I was inside with an electrician, who was also a longtime protestor and often carried a sign in front of nearby Planned Parenthood. He was about the same size. We are both bearded. Standing inside near the main doorway, looking up and checking the newly installed air conditioner for electrical problems, I looked out front just as a woman got out of an expensive SUV with a teenaged girl remaining in the car. The woman began to open our door. When she saw through the glass, two big, ugly, hairy men staring out at her, she let go of the door and turned away. Barbara came out and called out quietly, "We can help. Please come in." But the protestor (my electrician helper) overpowered Barbara's quiet words with his loud baritone, "Come in here. We don't do abortions." I stepped away from the door quickly. Barbara again called out, "Please come in. We can do a free pregnancy test." The woman, walking back to her car said, "I'm looking for Planned Parenthood." Our electrician then put the kibosh on any chance of saving the baby by saying loudly, "Don't go there. They're evil and they kill babies." Barbara's quiet, pleading words were drowned out by the stronger, deeper masculine voice and his bonehead words. The woman drove off and went next door. I immediately went out and told our sidewalk counselor, Peggy, about the two women and she spotted them just before they went in the abortionists' door. She called quietly to them without effect. The end of story was probably a dead baby and a mixed-up teen-ager, likely made worse.

What can CPC personnel learn from that story? One thing is that for many potential women clients, a man or men offers them no obvious help and probably frightens them. Another thing we again learn is that if we locate close to an abortion "clinic," many of their clients will mistakenly come to our door. We should be prepared for those women. We may be the Lord presenting the last chance for the woman and baby. Another thing we learn is that sometimes our well-meaning friends can flub our chance to save a baby.

What can the CPC leader do to offset that problem? Although that true story is an extreme case of bull-in-china-shop type (mis)counseling, there should be rules about the outside pray-ers and protestors staying away from the entrance and the waiting room of the CPC during abortion hours. Be aware of how we present ourselves to abortion minded clients. It is not deceitful to hide our religious and pro-life message until we can professionally present it in a calm, quiet counseling session. It is tactful and tactical for our mission.

There is a growing number of sidewalk counseling blogs available usually related to a church or from church oriented folks. I've seen sidewalk counseling information and videos from Catholic dioceses, Baptist churches, loose groups of Christians and other good folks, trying to increase the numbers of counselors and pray-ers at abortion facilities. Just Google "sidewalk counseling" and you'll find much good information. I hope the tide is turning. We need even more thoughtful baby-saving efforts at the abortion frontline.

What About Black and Latina Clients?

A shocking and unpublicized fact is that minority women (African-American and Hispanic) have 59 percent of all the abortions in America. Blacks and Hispanics tend to live in cities. Most free pregnancy centers are located in the suburbs or in small towns where few minorities live. The logical action for pro-lifers, trying to stop the evident genocide of our black and Hispanic pre-born babies is that we need to open centers or move existing centers into cities and very near where the abortionists are carrying out that genocide!

Having bi-lingual counselors (Spanish/English) at the CPC or on the frontline is very important. There are many other client ethnicities and languages and we need to communicate with them also. In Worcester, we have had clients from Ghana, Nigeria, Ivory Coast, Viet Nam, Haiti, Saudi Arabia, Thailand, El Salvador, Honduras, Canada, China, India, Guatemala, Mexico, Jamaica, Brazil, Egypt, Iran, Israel, Albania, Korea, Poland, Turkey, Greece, Russia, South Africa and many other nations. How are we able to provide translators for all those different people? We are not able. We just do the best we can, as you would with hand signals and Pidgin English. We pro-lifers love all the different colors of the babies and their mothers.

As I write this in May of 2010, I had an exhilarating experience last week. A former client from Ghana drove into Problem Pregnancy's parking lot in a late model SUV. Looking out the window, I asked Kathy, our major domo, "Who's that coming in?" She answered, "That's Efia. You haven't met her, but you have been writing checks for her monthly loan payment to the DCU (bank)." I remembered Efia (a pseudonym). She came to us, wanting an abortion and thinking we were Planned Parenthood. Our ultrasound showed that Efia was pregnant with twins. Kathy (God has given Kathy to us.) convinced Efia not to destroy the babies by offering her help with her difficult financial situation. Efia did not want to abort her babies, but saw no other option until she came to us. She was abandoned by the father of the babies and felt distraught and desperate. Efia had a well paid job and is an intelligent woman. She needed some initial financial help with her rent, but what she really needed was money to pay a monthly loan, until she could deliver the babies and then go back to work. Problem Pregnancy agreed to make that loan payment every month and did it for more than a year.

Now, to my exhilaration, Efia came into our office pushing a double stroller with two babies, one in tandem behind the other. Those two boys were the most beautiful babies, I have ever seen. They were four months old, husky with full heads of curly jet black hair, big onyx eyes full of life and curiosity, round, brown-sugar faces with big smiles and as healthy as babies can be. They looked like Mohammed Ali at four months old, multiplied by two. Those boys were world champions too and I had had a hand in saving their lives. There is no other exhilaration like that!

What about Converting "Clinic" Employees?

To any abortion clinic personnel reading these words, please consider my plea. We will help you leave your job. Even help financially, if possible. We will not judge you. If you need to speak to someone confidentially, I can be reached by emailing me at info@problempregnancy.org

In my 28 years of experience outside Planned Parenthood, I have never known for sure of any abortion facility employees who became pro-life and quit. But I have heard stories that were told to others about just such conversions. Planned Parenthood has a huge turnover of low-on-the-totem-pole employees. Some of Problem Pregnancy's volunteers develop friendly relationships with the security guard at the Worcester abortion site. One in particular, Mary B., is a very motherly woman. She's hard to resist.

A volunteer at a northeast pregnancy center recently confided to me, that the clinic manager of the abortion facility adjacent to his CPC, hates what she does for living. While she is searching for another job, she is steering many of her abortion-minded clients surreptitiously to the pro-life organization.

Those abortion "clinic" employees, involved in "counseling" for abortions, assisting at abortions or otherwise facilitating abortions, can't avoid the reality and the horror. The new ultrasound scanners are so clear that the abortionist and assistants see the truth every day—that a real baby is being killed. Abortionists don't allow clients to see the ultra-sound scanner with its clear evidence, that there is a real baby. After 14-weeks gestation, the fetus could not be recognized as anything but a tiny baby. This takes an emotional toll on doctors, nurses and aides in the abortion business, according to a Weekly Standard article, "Mugged by Ultra-sound" by Jon Shields (January 2010).

This revulsion of seeing cut up human babies seems to affect only a minority of these accomplices to defect, Shields reports. Most continue in their "work." Dilation and evacuation" (D and E) abortions are the most common, second trimester method and considered "safer" for the mother. There have been millions of D and E abortions in the U.S.A., according to Shields.

This method has the doctor dilate (expand) the woman's cervix and with a cold set of stainless forceps, he then digs into the woman's most private and vulnerable organs and pulls apart the "fetus." Distress at the very least, for the abortionist must be a result of such a horror. Abortionists Warren Hern and Billie Corrigan found that although their staff members "approved of second trimester abortion in principle," there "were few positive comments about D and E itself." According to Hern and Corrigan, reactions included "shock, dismay, amazement, disgust, fear, and sadness." Other studies confirmed Hern and Corrigan's results, finding strong emotional reactions during or following the procedures and employees' disquieting dreams. In other words, abortion "clinic" personnel are human.

Another study showed that abortion staff was upset at seeing a "fetus" die; regardless of how committed they were to abortion. It seems that no amount of ideology can overcome negative emotional reactions to abortion. Dr. Paul

Jarrett, was one of the first abortion doctors to quit and after only 23 abortions. In 1974 he performed an abortion on a baby at 14 weeks, "As I brought out the rib cage, I looked and saw a tiny, beating heart. And when I found the head of the baby, I looked squarely in the face of another human being—a human being that I just killed."

An American Life League associate, who was formerly an employee at a Planned Parenthood clinic, found that disposing of fetal bodies as medical waste was more than she could bear. Soon after leaving her job, she described her experiences. "No one at Planned Parenthood wanted this job. I had to look at the tiny hands and feet. There were times when I wanted to cry." She was persuaded to quit by a pro-life protester outside her clinic.

A current director of a CPC, Kathy Sparks has a similar story about her time as an abortion mill employee. She was responsible for disposing of fetal remains. She reports on the Pro-Life Action League website, "The baby's bones were far too developed to rip them up with [the doctor's] curette, so he had to pull the baby out with forceps. He brought out three or four major pieces. I took the baby to the clean up room, I set him down and I began weeping uncontrollably. I cried and cried. This little face was perfectly formed." She quit the next day.

Another converted pro-lifer and now Operation Rescue volunteer was formerly a secretary for George Tiller, a former, late term Kansas abortionist. After her first time being involved in taking dead babies to Tiller's crematorium, she quit her job. Abby Johnson, the former director of a Dallas Planned Parenthood, quit after viewing an ultrasound scan of an unborn baby being suctioned out of its mother's womb. Johnson is now a speaker at many pro-life affairs.

Dr. Bernard Nathanson is the most famous abortionist to be converted by ultrasound technology. In the early 1970s, Nathanson was the largest abortion provider in the Western world. He performed more than 60 thousand abortions, including one on his own child. He has written a book, "Aborting America" and produced a film, "The Silent Scream," a documentary of an ultrasound abortion that showed the fetus trying to avoid dismemberment. There is even a new Spanish language play written of his conversion.

Carol Everett is another well known pro-lifer, who once ran an abortion business in Texas. Today she rues the 35 thousand abortions done in her "clinic." She speaks at many pro-life dinners and tells of the many abortions done on non-pregnant women, just for the money. Although the majority of clinic workers remain committed to the pro-abortion cause, sidewalk counselors and others on the frontline should pray for these people, be kind to them and if given an opportunity, try to win them over to the right side.

* * *

Problem Pregnancy has counselors, who have had abortions. One (J.) is active in Silent No More, an organization of women, who regret their abortions. They are very good in client sessions, because they have lived it and know what they are talking about. We are fortunate to get these strong, determined women, healing from abortion, as counselors.

Problem Pregnancy does special classes for Sunday school classes of teenagers. Those kids see a real (married) mother getting an ultrasound. They are amazed by the baby moving around in the womb. The piece de resistance, however, is the last session when one of our counselors, who has had a previous abortion, speaks to the students about her horrific abortion experiences. Their eyes are opened. We repeatedly hear them saying as they leave, regarding the obvious life of an unborn baby, "How come we never hear about that at school?"

9.

Fundraising

Every non-profit needs to raise money or go out of business. Most pregnancy centers were founded by social worker types and often the business end is not the founder's strong suit. Experience at running a business or at fundraising is scant at those CPCs. If an experienced fundraising person could be recruited to volunteer at such a social worker-run CPC, it would allow the founder to concentrate on the main event—saving babies. From my experience, the need for business experience at pregnancy centers is evident. Volunteers, experienced in business, are in short supply.

Fundraising is an art not a science, but it grows out of good business practices, like planning, targeting markets, aggressive sales and marketing, good printed materials, development, regular follow up, good bookkeeping and common sense.

Next to God and volunteers, money is the most important thing in running a non-profit agency. Pregnancy centers need small amounts or large amounts of money, depending on their agenda and their mission. Even the smallest group needs funds for postage stamps, newspaper ads, office equipment, brochures, utilities, seed money for fundraisers, etc. How do they raise those funds?

Some of us old timers know how to do that. We are not frightened by large money problems. We have been involved with profit-making organizations and understand the most effective methods to get things done. A business oriented veteran would not be fazed by the need to raise $30 thousand annually for a small local CPC or $200 thousand for a mid-range CPC. Business type volunteers are sorely needed in this baby-saving effort, because other volunteers do not know how to effectively raise money.

Fundraising Methods

There are many different ways that non-profits raise money. I know of only a few that would provide enough funds to organize and run a new CPC Plus facility next to an abortion mill. The center with which I have been involved, uses one or more of the following methods to raise money. Some of the following methods would not produce enough funds for our project.

Pot Luck Suppers

Pot luck suppers, usually held once a year, are almost always a high profit fundraising event, but only if the speaker doesn't charge a fee and if the supper site is free. The organization's volunteers invite friends and new potential supporters to the free supper. The volunteer not only brings the audience, she buys the food and perhaps the wine. She cooks a casserole, for example, and maybe a home baked pie to be served at the her sponsored table. The event requires an interesting pro-life speaker. If he is well known, all the better. The organization provides free coffee and soft drinks. After the supper, the organization's leader or the dinner speaker exhorts the crowd for donations. The table volunteer collects the cash, checks and pledges, records them and hands them over to the organization. I have been at Pot Luck Suppers that have brought in $5 thousand and more, net.

Baby Showers

Many churches will run a baby shower around Advent or Mothers Day for Problem Pregnancy. We really love baby showers, because our clients constantly need so many of the shower gifts. Things like diapers, car seats, baby wipes, onesies, baby outfits, baby oil, talcum, hand knitted hats, booties, sweaters, and baby blankets are constantly needed by our mothers and babies. Our cellar is full of those items after the baby shower season. We usually do not need to buy such items throughout the whole year, because our churches are so generous. Sometimes there will be a few checks but baby showers are not really fundraisers. They are very welcome however.

What about Appeal Letters?

Appeal letters are a tried and true method of consistently raising funds. Problem Pregnancy's main source of funds comes from four appeal letters that I write at strategic times during the calendar year. Such letters are not "newsletters." Newsletters are not intended to raise money. They are intended to keep supporters up to date with the organization's events and efforts. Some non-profit people think that newsletters will raise money, but they are wrong, even though a few donations may result. A good friend and a Problem Pregnancy supporter, who spent 40 years in the advertising business, had an appropriate expression, "An all purpose letter is a no purpose letter." A Russian homily applies also, "Chase two rabbits. Catch none." The appeal letter's purpose is to raise funds for the CPC. Nothing else. It should be written carefully so it immediately catches the attention of the reader. It should then tell an interesting story, related to the work of the organization. It should ask for funds at least twice within the text and then really press hard at the end for money. A well written, appeal letter will extract donations from old supporters and new supporters. Anecdotes about real hard cases and the saving of babies with pseudonym names and lots of drama, really work. All such mailings should request donations. There also should be a donor coupon and a reply envelope if you want a high return.

One thing that donors like is lean non-profits. Under the "Saving Babies at Calvary" section above, I recommend starting or running an all-volunteer organization with no payroll. Dedicated volunteers saving babies without pay have lots of credibility when asking for funds.

Another key to receiving a good return from your mailed appeal letters is that it should be sent to a good mailing list. How is that accomplished? Most of your original donors will be your own volunteers, their friends and your relatives during your early days. Begin your list with them. Tough it out for a year and work on building your mailing list. There must be one person who is the volunteer fundraiser. I am that person at Problem Pregnancy. He or she will need a donor database software program. It should be relatively simple to use. This database should be independent of the client tracking database. I use an older version of Filemaker Pro. The designated fundraiser should continually pester all the volunteers to give him names and addresses of potential donors. He should get lists of local Protestant and Catholic clergy and religious (religious are Catholic monks, nuns, brothers and other consecrated folks) and add them to the database. He should read all the local newspapers, secular and church related, especially the letters to the editor to find sympathetic, potential donors to add. Sometimes he will know a last name and a city but no address. This website, www.whitepages.com/5175 (Switchboard) has been very helpful in finding addresses and phone numbers if all I have is a name and town. I have begun adding email addresses when I can get them. Another idea is to think about a possible recent statewide referendum that would have brought out pro-family voters. Such a digital voting list would be free from the Secretary of State's office. Many of those voters would be pro-life and likely to donate to a good baby-saving CPC. Using this method plus begging small lists from churches and other friendly organizations and with some other more creative ideas, I have built an 18 thousand-person mailing list. It is a daily effort to do this and keep it up to date. Mailing four appeal letters to that list each year provides enough funds to operate our Worcester, Massachusetts pregnancy resource center and sidewalk counseling effort. Early in our history, we did the dinner; bake sale, raffle and walk kind of fundraising events. We no longer do those things. The return is too small for the effort. To get some ideas about appeal letters, I have provided a few of my Problem Pregnancy letters in the Appendix.

Emails and Website Appeals

There are some non-profits using email solicitations to raise funds. I'm skeptical about the success of such campaigns. I use the web, sending and receiving emails constantly, but I don't think I ever responded to a request for money from an email. In order to do so, the donor must stop what he is doing on the net, go find his checkbook, an envelope and a stamp and then write a check, find the correct address, etc. It is inconvenient and I think it will not work well. Maybe there will be a convenient way in the future but I don't see email fundraising yet as a viable method.

On the other hand, using your non-profit's website, with a credit card payment system to collect the donations, does work. The hard work is to get the potential donor to the charity's website where the pitch is made for the gift. I think that the internet will become more effective in the future for all non-profits.

Baby Bottles

Although I have never used the Baby Bottle fund-raising method, I understand that other groups have been quite successful with it. It works best with supportive churches. With the pastor's permission and a parish layperson in charge, real plastic baby bottles are distributed to church members, who individually fill them at home with change or bills. It is usually done during Lent or another specific time period. A secondary benefit to the charity would be the addition of the baby bottle donors' names and addresses to the CPC's mailing list. I know a maternity home that brings in a substantial amount of its annual income from its well-planned Baby Bottle program.

What is "Planned Giving"?

I think of Planned Giving and Large Giver personal appeal efforts, as two different methods but I am going to cover them together, because they are related. They complement each other actually. Planned Giving is a very trendy development tool to raise funds. It is used mostly by large charities, which have paid development officers. Some of those people actually went to college to study how to raise money for non-profits. Would you believe that?

I am constantly invited with other "development officers" to seminars by experts on Planned Giving. An intelligent volunteer fundraiser does this kind of fundraising instinct-ively, but in a smaller way. The way a small organization would do Planned Giving follows. Let us say a small non-profit has an active supporter, who donates irregularly but generously. The designated fundraiser would look for an opportunity to see the donor in a social setting, after Mass or at a social event, for instance. If the fundraiser could get the conversation going in the right direction, she might thank the donor, tell him how the organization is doing and then tell the donor about the new automatic credit card monthly withdrawal program. If he likes the idea—voila!– planned giving. Another fund raising idea would be to ask a large donor, who gives irregularly to send one larger gift annually. When I do that, I suggest to the donor, that a reminder letter would be sent and then ask what part of the year should the reminder arrive, related to his financial situation and taxes. Both of these are planned giving, lower case.

What the big charities do is identify and target market the potential big donors and then try to find someone on their own board, who knows one or more of them. The idea is that the board member would call or otherwise contact the target and gush about the wonderful cause with which he is involved. The board member would then "rat-out" the potential donor to the development officer. The development person would then call the target donor and set up a face-to-face. He or she then does what my sainted father would call, "putting the arm on him." The professional development people describe it more genteelly. They call it personal solicitation. Mailings, emailings, websites and other non-personal contacts are not nearly as effective as "putting the arm on" a large donor. Large donors need to know that their gifts are not wasted on silly things. The pro-life donor needs to know that, without his donation, babies will die. Do not be afraid to tell him that, but only if it is true.

Development people are salesmen in pink camouflage (They are usually women). She will identify her market, plan a sales and marketing program and then go out and make the sale or in this case get the donation. Small local charities should follow her example and do the same. Volunteers are perfectly able to do that, but in a much smaller arena. Sometimes a designated volunteer is a novice and is nervous about asking for appointments with potential large donors. Most of us would rather send an impersonal letter asking for funds instead of personally seeing a possible donor and "hitting him up." But in real business, most new accounts come from a salesman's persistence, his passion and his presentation of his company's products. Being in front of your target allows you read his responses. Are you asking for too large an amount? Are you asking for too little? Watch his face. Like a poker player, you look for "tells." Read him and listen to his comments and you will know how to tailor your "ask."

There are many reasons why meeting people face to face is valuable. I think there is no question that personal contact is the most effective way to get the result that you want. I'm going to focus on why it is sometimes difficult for volunteers to ask for that donor appointment—the fear factor. The fear derives from not knowing what to say or how to respond to your possible donor's objections. The fear of being thought ridiculous or the fear of hearing that nasty word—*no*.

Practicing beforehand on a colleague will help make those personal meetings go better. Try out your responses to possible objections. Getting negative answers is part of the selling business and the fund-raising business. In past incarnations, I have been a sales manager and my advice to my salesmen was that selling is a numbers game. If you make 30 sales calls, you will get one sale on average. That average is for certain cold call selling. I do not know the numbers average in fundraising. You would probably vet your potential donors in advance, so that your face-to-face visits would be more successful than cold call selling. The *no* sales should be many fewer in fundraising. You will get better as you gain experience and the more experience you have, the easier it will be in dealing with your fear factor.

Just as salesmen have trepidation when the time rolls around for a follow up telephone call to close the potential customer, the fundraiser also has that fear about her donor. Will that target say no? Was he offended by my previous "ask"? We all have negative thinking to overcome. You will wonder if the potential donor will think that you are pestering him? Remember, it is not you, to which the donor would give his money. It's the pregnancy resource center and the endangered babies and their mothers who receive his contributions. So pester away!

Persistence is always a good thing and never a bad thing. I developed an attitude very early in my 50-year sales career, that shows up in my initial presentation and my follow-up calls. That attitude says non-verbally the following to my potential customer or donor, "I have spent much of my time, money and effort to present you with the reasons why you should buy my product or donate to my cause. I deserve and expect to get a timely answer, either yes or no." Fundraisers should not be afraid to develop that attitude or even say it outright, if the potential donor dithers too much, even if it seems embarrassing. In sales, as in fundraising, follow up, follow up, follow up are three of the keys for success. Large donors need to be handled professionally, like the potential sale that they are.

Our organization uses large donors to do large things. Buying our building, buying our ultrasound unit, replacing the roof, special advertising programs and paying for signage are some of those big things paid for by large donors.

Bake Sales and Other Fundraising Methods

There are other methods used by non-profits to raise money. I do not think they are as good as some of the ones listed above. I know that creative people can do wonders with seemingly mundane fundraising schemes. For instance I was recently told by a woman who is a bake sale expert that a large bake sale, organized correctly and held at a church on a Sunday, would bring in $1,000 or more every time and all the goodies would be sold. Perhaps others know how to make car washes, yard sales and raffles more lucrative also. There are other events that require a particular kind of fundraising person to be effective; e.g. golf tournaments, walks for life or runs for life. Membership dues can add a little to the bottom line but unless your organization has a huge membership, it will not replace the necessary large fundraising programs.

Foundations

Most contributions to CPCs are from individuals, who agree with the baby-saving and women-helping goals. Centers also receive funds from churches, church groups, other pro-life groups, some companies, a few services agencies and some foundations.

Recently I had a meeting with a group of good Catholic pro-lifers who were concerned about the large number of unborn babies being killed in Massachusetts. They were considering opening a CPC to save some of those babies. I was there as an unpaid consultant to answer their questions, regarding the current abortion "clinic" scenario within Massachusetts. My friend, Chris Slattery of Emergency

Mother Care (EMC) in New York attended, as an expert also. These people were older and had no experience at running CPCs or at sidewalk counseling. They were, however, substantial folks with varied business and life experiences. Chris and I were of the same mind toward the end of the meeting. We suggested that they start a foundation that specialized in grants to new and existing CPCs. In other words, they could save many babies by funding the baby-savers. We thought that such a foundation would aid struggling Massachusetts pregnancy centers. That idea had the added benefit of using the many talents of that group. Perhaps that idea will come to fruition.

There is another IRS entity called Supporting Organizations (509(a)(3) that is similar to a foundation but without as much IRS oversight. That structure is tax exempt by supporting tax exempt charities. Worth a look.

There may be readers, who like the foundation idea for their state or city. The need is great. The biggest need is to provide funds for CPCs to buy or lease property nearby abortion facilities, presently unimpeded. Advertising money to compete with the abortionists' high budget promotions is a real need for many struggling CPCs. The abortionists like Planned Parenthood earn huge profits by killing babies. They then use those profits to advertise to get more "business" and more babies to kill. The more successful the abortionist is in aborting babies, the more money he has to advertise. Pregnancy centers on the other hand spend contributors' money to provide free services to pregnant mothers. The more successful the pregnancy center is in saving babies, the more it costs CPCs. It isn't fair, but it is true. Elsewhere in this book I mention that at least one state (Minnesota) is providing grants to pregnant women for material needs. This is lowering that state's rate of abortion. Also the federal government *may* be doing something like that. What is needed is private money put into pro-life foundations. Dedicated foundations throughout the U.S.A., providing grants to CPCs for practical aid to clients is one way to put a thumb on the scale of justice to even things out a little.

Stewardship of Donors' Money

New and existing CPC leaders need at least basic skills in financial management. Do not hand off that responsibility. You will be asking for trouble. Things like cash management and bookkeeping need continuous attention and integrity. Funds come to my center, almost always in checks by mail after an appeal letter. I use a simple Quicken bookkeeping software program and a Filemaker Pro database to record each donation by amount, date, name and address. Every single donor gets a mailed, personal thank you. The database allows me to let larger contributors know at tax filing time, if requested, the amount of their annual total. Quicken allows me to keep a running tab on the income and outgo and the comparison between this year and last year's totals. It also provides an annual record for our accountant at the May 15 tax filing time. Even though we are tax exempt, the IRS and state tax people require non-profit corporations to file.

Conflicts of interest should be avoided. Personal or professional interests of insiders are not always in the best interest of the CPC. Despite that concern, I try to find supportive, paid pro-lifers, to do the outside work, not performed by volunteers. Things like; snowplowing, electrical work or maintenance should be contracted to trusted pro-lifers, if possible. Often we get the best price from those friendly vendors. I know that public perception is important and any misunderstanding should be explained. Be careful of even the appearance of impropriety. Honesty and good business practices will prevail in this important part of being a leader.

Raising funds from donors has another side to it. The treasurer or other person responsible for the organization's money must be very careful of how the funds are spent. Even more careful than spending his own dollars. The pregnancy center's funds are held in trust. It is the babies' money. It is the donors' money.

Most of the funds spent at Problem Pregnancy are for necessary expenses like mortgage payments, heat, electric, phone, etc. There is sometimes discretionary spending, using money left over, after the necessary spending. Not an ordinary thing but we welcome it when it happens. The CPC leader always has more projects in line for that money than money to use.

I've mentioned above how we save babies by paying for the urgent, ancillary needs of our pregnant, abortion minded clients. This spending requires the leader to put a different hat on. When I do it, I become, not Santa Claus but the Grinch. There are clients, who will try to defraud us. Some clients will invent colorful tales of dire needs, when they know money is available. A friend once used this expression, which I like, "People are funny with money."

We have established policies so that we limit the possibility of fraud. All payments to clients or to vendors of clients must go through two of Problem Pregnancy's board members. We never give cash, always a check. Our assumption is that the client will ask for more than is necessary. I'm the final authority and I'm one of those two board members. We don't write checks to any clients but only to the landlords, child care establishments, banks or other vendors. I personally call the vendors to check out each client's story. We know that many babies are saved, when we provide practical and sometimes expensive solutions. We are very careful with our donors' dollars. It's my opinion that our policy of paying out real money for an abortion minded pregnant woman's needs does indeed save babies' lives. I think the same needs to be done at every CPC in the land, but done carefully. The small risk of client fraud is overwhelmed by the likelihood of saving a real girl or boy from being chopped up.

My Secret Fundraising Method

Now I'm going to divulge my most secret and productive fundraising method – tattoo parlors. I've got a network of 15 thousand tattoo parlors across the U.S.A. ready to kick back 50 percent of all the pro-life tattoos put on senior citizen pro-lifers. There are three conditions. One that the tattoo must read: "Tattooed for Life." Two, in order to get the most publicity for our baby-saving cause, we need face-time on the street. Therefore the tat must be positioned onto the forehead, centered above the eyebrows. For those old folks who are eyebrow challenged, the tattooist will use the geezer's runny nose as a centering point. And the third condition involves the new brighter inks available for tattoos now. In order to get the CPC donation, the tattoo inks used must be neon green and red. The special curmudgeon price will be $150 with $75 going to your CPC. The tattoo shops will also be skimming a little as my cut (pun intended) for coming up with this great fundraising idea.

Seriously now folks, I actually know of a tattoo shop owner who organized his fellow downtown businessmen to stop Planned Parenthood from moving into his Massachusetts city. Coming soon to a seedy neighborhood near you the next big, popular fad – "Tattooed for Life" forehead tattoos!

10.

Volunteers

There are many kinds of volunteers. The questionnaire below is used by a Catholic oriented CPC to winnow out potential volunteer counselors who would not be in sync with its "Gospel of Life" philosophy.

Questionnaire for Volunteer Counselors

Name_____Phone_____

1. How did you hear about us?
2. What do you know about us?
3. Why do you want to volunteer here?
4. How many hours a week are you able to commit? (Minimum 2 hrs. per week)
5. How do you feel about abortion? Do you ever feel that it is right in certain situations?
6. Have you always felt abortion was wrong?
7. Have you ever had an abortion? Do you have any friend or family members who have had abortions?
8. Do you practice a faith? If so, what faith?
9. Your feelings about artificial birth control?
10. Your feelings about natural family planning?
11. Your position about premarital sex? Abstinence and chastity—Are you comfortable promoting these?

* * *

In order for this dream of mine to be fulfilled, American CPCs will need very good volunteers. Although the task needs more women than men volunteers, we need plenty of both. For this life-saving task, we need volunteers of all ages and stripes.

Older Volunteers

I am irritated by so-called experts on the subject of aging Americans in the 21st Century. Most of it is drivel. One expert's theory posits that our previous lives will define our last years here on terra firma. In other words, if life was not kind to you during your childhood, youth, or adulthood, if you were not a big success in business or if you made consequential mistakes in your past life, then you will be bound to repeat that bad routine in your dotage. That is a pile of warm horsebuns! Sure, we can't fix our less than perfect earlier lives, but we can certainly build new lives starting today. That should be easier now that our children have grown and our responsibilities have probably lessened. I disagree with that predestination expert. There really can be *A Second Act*. We can do what we damn well please. Most of us geezers have more freedom now and we could choose to live our remaining years in a moral, decent manner or in indolence, no matter how we spent the first three quarters of our lives.

My grandpa years are being spent doing much of what I did in my adult years. Childhood is a time of instruction when we learn. Adulthood is a time of intelligence but old

151

age is supposed to be a time of wisdom. I think that old age is the last chance for us to be led by the Lord. Take that last chance, my fellow old timers.

In order to be so led by the Lord, each of us needs to further develop the Cardinal Virtues—prudence, temperance, justice and fortitude. Although, as we age some of our internal demons get easier to handle, we still need to regularly bludgeon the Seven Deadly Sins in our life; pride, avarice, lust, envy, gluttony, anger and sloth.

At this time of our lives, some might balk at the idea of giving ourselves to a great moral cause like saving babies at an abortion facility. There is a phenomenon that I have observed in my long sales career. The prospective buyer most negative to your sales pitch is often the customer who is closest to buying and is afraid to hear more of your sales pitch because he might succumb and end up buying. The indifferent prospective customer is not a likely buyer but the buyer who tells you loudly not to bug him is often a good candidate for a sale. So maybe you, the potential volunteer candidate making the most negative noise about not joining up might be the one most likely to sign up as a baby-saver.

At whatever age, we must consider ethics in volunteer work. I have often had to examine my motives for offering to do a volunteer job. Am I getting something of value personally from this job? Am I avoiding something that I should be doing at home or in my business and this non-profit job is giving me an excuse not to do it? Am I really looking to get publicity or atta-boys, if I do this job? It is in that vein, that each of us must examine our conscience regarding our motives. Even we ancients must face our sinfulness and understand that even today in our old age, our actions and our reactions could be related to our own sinful nature. So joining a CPC Plus and beginning to do God's work, will help us to bludgeon our internal demons further.

Give respect to the old—Leviticus 19:32. I agree with this bible verse but as an old man, I do not ask for respect. I expect respect for what I do. I have changed very little from what I was 20 years ago when I was a chirpy 51. I work every day. I spend countless hours volunteering. I maintain my properties. I am active at local, state and national politics. I go to Mass every Sunday and on holy days and I help at my parish. The difference is that I have more aches and maladies and I'd like a nap once a day. Also, I have a little less energy than I used to have. Why should I need to ask for respect? There are so many younger people wasting their time on meaningless games, reading People Magazine, stupidly trying to beat overwhelming odds at casinos and spending hours looking at inane TV shows. They are the ones that need to beg for respect, not me.

Problem Pregnancy, our pregnancy center has been blessed for 28 years with wonderful loving and caring women volunteers. Hundreds of them! Without our women counselors, inside and outside, no babies would have been saved and no mothers helped. Problem Pregnancy has saved thousands of babies. All the other information about running a CPC, written in this book, is useless without those selfless women who volunteer to do a very tough job. I love them all and God loves them too. I know it.

Rates of volunteering vary widely from state to state, but whatever state they call home, volunteers are more likely to be women than men. Surprisingly women with children and women who work have a higher volunteer rate than other women. Those are among the findings of "Volunteering in America: State Trends and Rankings," a first ever federal study by the Corporation for National and Community Service. Across the country, 32 percent of women volunteer, compared with 25 percent of men. A previous federal study, in 1974, found that women volunteered more than men do, but that employed women accounted for only 43 percent of female volunteers, with 54 percent of the volunteers outside the workforce.

By 2005, those numbers were reversed with 63 percent of female volunteers employed and 34 percent outside the labor force. Females volunteer at significantly higher rates than do males in every state. Women with children under age 18 volunteer at a significantly higher rate (40 percent), than women without young children (29 percent). The role of women with children who volunteer is particularly important, because of the impact their volunteering has on their children. Another study released in November 2005 revealed that youth coming from families where their parents and/or siblings volunteer are more likely to volunteer themselves.

28 percent of American adults volunteered in 2005, an increase of nearly six million volunteers since 2002. In 2005 Americans spent a median of 50 hours per year volunteering, and gave a total of 8.2 billion hours of volunteer service. According to Independent Sector, the estimated dollar value of all American volunteers' time equated to a value of $147.6 billion dollars in 2005.

The typical American volunteer is a white female who gives 50 hours per year volunteering through a religious organization. Why do women volunteer? There are many reasons. Women volunteer to make social contacts and expand their sense of community. Women like to be with other women who have similar interests. Women are hardwired to be engaged in their communities. Volunteering connects women. They share, they compare and they adopt new strategies to make a difference in the world—their world. They volunteer because they get back more than they give. Women feel better about everything, because they become part of something bigger than themselves. Hooray for women!

Men Volunteers

Why don't men volunteer? There are many social service agencies, that are not able to recruit male volunteers and they fret about it, often in writing. Some of the fretting from such women administrators are typical gobbledy-gook social worker speak. Non-profit administrators worry about the lack of men volunteers. Possible causes mentioned are the unfortunate worries men have about machismo, their gender roles, their inability to take a ribbing from male peers for doing "women's" work or the fear of men being unfairly thought of as a child predator if the charity involves children.

Other concerns of men, according the female leaders of some non-profits, are the following; that men think that the job isn't important enough for them or that it doesn't provide enough action or that it is too "feminine" for them or that the job will become permanent or that they are not ready for such a commitment. All these concerns have some legitimacy, I think. There is also an opinion that women are socialized to be nurturers and helpers but men are not. I think both genders believe that and it is most often true. Society expects men to be independent, aggressive, and strong. Nurturing, however, may not be a required quality or even asked for in many volunteer positions.

Some men's natural characteristics, such as independence, actually would help to make a good volunteer. Regardless of the truth about the male ability to nurture and males' obligation to earn money, the fact that these perceptions exist reveals stereotypes that may deter men from volunteering. Despite NOW and Ms Magazine, men and women believe that men and women have different roles and capabilities in life and that includes in volunteering

Any prospective volunteer needs to be invited, man or woman. Some just have never got into the habit of volunteering. Some men need to be horsed a little to make that initial phone call, expressing an interest in volunteering. Sometimes a little effort on the agency's part may be the whack upside the head that a man needs, to start volunteering. Easy access to volunteering may help a lot.

Even more important for attracting men volunteers is that there be goals and targets. Men need concrete illustrations about what benchmarks can be reached by volunteers. That would scratch a guy's itch for competition. In other words, how much money did you raise today? How many babies did you save this morning? A man's ability to assess his progress and to assign quantitative values to his effectiveness is all important to male volunteers. What did I get done today? Hooray for men!

Where are the Young Volunteers?

Recent national polls have been good news for pro-lifers. For example, the Gallup poll asks the same question year after year, "With respect to the abortion issue, would you consider yourself to be pro-choice or pro-life?" The latest (June 2010) poll shows that Americans are pro-life over pro-choice by 2 percent. Since the November 2006 Gallup poll that asked the same question, the change has gone from 10 percent down to 2 percent up for the pro-life side, an astounding 12 percent increase in less than four years. This change seems to be even more pronounced within the younger population and even further weighted within the young woman population. Pro-abortion groups are publicly wringing their hands, reflecting their concern about this since our youth become our leaders very quickly. Pro-lifers should be pleased with all of these data.

In April 2010 Nancy Keenan, president of NARAL said about the huge turnout of young folks at the January 2010

March for Life in Washington, "I just thought, my gosh, they are so young. There are so many of them, and they are so young." She also confessed that she considers herself part of the "postmenopausal militia." I have been told by witnesses that about half of the 2010 marchers appeared to be younger than thirty.

I hope all the good news is true. Our final victory will be indicated by strong involvement of young people in every category of pro-life work. So far I have not seen much evidence that young people are volunteering at CPCs or maternity homes. So far these fired-up young people are not writing letters to the editor or Op Ed pieces either. I feel like St. Thomas. Metaphorically I want to stick my hand into the wounds so I can believe.

Historically Problem Pregnancy gets almost no young volunteers. Worcester has ten colleges. Once in a while a Holy Cross College or Assumption College student will train as a counselor. We have had college pro-life groups invite us to speak or run baby showers for us. We have a few rare young folks who have been very helpful volunteers. That young volunteer is even scarcer today. I have discussed this with other leaders of different kinds of pro-life groups. They are hopeful but like us they do not see many young volunteers. Why? Where are our young folks? We need them.

11.

Religion

In this chapter, I will discuss the various ways that religion intertwines itself within the pro-life movement and in particular into crisis pregnancy centers.

Who Are Our Friends?

In the next chapter I will describe, who is the enemy of the millions of aborted babies and of the pro-life movement. In this section of the Religion Chapter, I will discuss who are our religious friends. There are many disparate pro-lifers with no groupings, and there are also groups, that are known to be pro-life. Of course, the Roman Catholic Church has been and still is a heroic leader against the legalization of abortion and other protection of human life issues. The Southern Baptist Church, the Eastern Orthodox Church, the Mormons, the Assembly of God Church, many of the urban black churches and many independent Evangelical churches are also stalwarts for the anti-abortion movement. The Orthodox Jews are often pro-life and Muslims are supposed to be also, but those last two religious groups are much more careful and quiet about their support.

The national Republican establishment, although not a religious group, is publicly pro-life, since the 1976 National

Convention Platform. I was a delegate to that convention in Kansas City. I was part of a real donnybrook between the country club GOP and the new ethnic, religious and southern Republicans, who won at least with the platform. Unfortunately, we lost when Ronald Reagan came within a whisker of beating President Jerry Ford for the nomination. The country club Republicans are still pro-abortion but the national party is pro-life.

There are quasi-religious bodies that are strong in their support of pro-life causes like radio and TV entities; e.g. Dr. James Dobson's "Focus on the Family," Eternal Word Television Network (EWTN), National Pro-Life Radio, CatholicTV and many other Christian and Catholic radio and TV stations.

Surprisingly there are members of the enemy team who have broken with their groups and are supporters of pro-life causes; e.g., Libertarians for Life; Episcopalians for Life, Feminists for Life, the Pro-Life Alliance of Gays and Lesbians and the most unusual, the Atheist and Agnostic Pro-Life League. Those are some of our friends.

Catholic and Evangelical Pro-Lifers

In 1973 about the same time as the Roe v. Wade Supreme Court decision exploded onto the U.S.A., there was an evolving political power change happening. Catholics were moving up the social and economic ladder quickly. In Boston that meant that Yankee Republican (read Protestant) elected officials were being replaced by Catholic ones (read Democrat). Yet vestiges of the previous segregation by religion lingered. Since most of the pro-abortion leaders were Protestant or Jewish, many Catholics thought that all Protestants wanted to abort little babies. Most of the Protestant secular leaders were supportive of the Roe v. Wade decision. Therefore it was my opinion at the time that the Yankees thought that abortion would be a good thing. Abortion would decrease the number of babies, born to the large Catholic families and perhaps give political power back to the infertile Yankees. I still think that Massachusetts Yankees at that time believed that.

The pro-life movement began in that religious ferment, at least in Boston and I think also in the rest of New England and probably much of the Northeast too. After Roe there was a loud national response that was almost 100 percent Roman Catholic. The horror of Roe was handed down to America by a Supreme Court of whom the majority was Protestant and written by Justice Harry Blackmun, a Methodist. Catholics were still wary of Protestants. After a few years, some of the Evangelical Protestants began to speak out against abortion and to organize. Catholic pro-lifers were very happy about that. We needed allies. That was the beginning of a real ecumenism, rather than the previous, hot air version where clerics of different faiths attended each other's services and made happy-talk and parroted torrents of feel-good inanities.

Two Different Anti-Abortion Philosophies

There are at least two different philosophies, regarding the purpose of the pro-life movement. One philosophy says that the primary purpose is to save babies' lives from abortion. The other philosophy says that the purpose of the pro-life movement is the conversion of pregnant mothers' hearts and therefore the changing of the culture, leading to the end of abortion. These two approaches play out in the management of CPCs. Most centers operated by Roman Catholics work to save babies first and then when the baby is safe, try to change the mothers' hearts. Most centers, run by Evangelicals, think their primary job is to convert the client to Jesus Christ and to whatever church is managing the pregnancy center.

There is a national association of pregnancy centers that adheres to Evangelical principles. In its website under "The Hope of Pregnancy Centers" are the following words. "The ultimate aim of . . . and its network of pregnancy centers is to share the love and truth of Jesus Christ in both word and deed. As a result, the hearts of women and men are being changed by Christ's love to desire positive and healthy choices. In addition, those struggling with past abortions are finding God's healing and forgiveness." Although its web site's vision statement includes a short passage of concern for life of the unborn baby, the stress is on the mother. I have mixed feeling in criticizing any of my colleagues but I think this focus is on the wrong person. Its website gives short shrift to unborn babies. The pregnant woman's heart and soul is their focus. I disagree with that direction. All CPCs should be concerned with the mother and of course, working with the mother often saves the baby. But the innocent baby, about to be killed, should be the raison d'etre. Nothing else!

* * *

The Christian Action Council (CAC) was an early Evangelical anti-abortion incarnation. It was founded in 1975 by Dr. Harold O.J. Brown with influences from Dr. C. Everett Koop and Boston Evangelical leader Dr. Francis Schaeffer. In the early days, I was friendly with one of CAC's early organizers, Reverend John Rankin. The two different types of Christian pro-lifers (Catholic and Evangelical) figuratively tiptoed around each other in those early years. Even today I need to take off my RC Donegal tweed scally cap and put on my Evangelical bible college baseball cap when I work with my Christian fellows on joint projects.

The people working in the pro-life movement, whether Catholic or Evangelical, are very devout Christians, but our denominations' natural demeanors are different. Evangelicals use biblical references often even in everyday conversation, while Catholics are more secular, even racy in their ordinary repartee. Another sticking point is that many Evangelicals think that everyone else is not "saved," whereas Catholics believe that they have the one true and the original Christian church. Catholics get quite angry, when an Evangelical asks, "Do you have a personal relationship with Christ?" Those things cause members of both groups to bristle. Our differences like thorny brambles remain between us. Although we Catholics welcomed our pro-life Christian brothers and sisters, we remained wary and tried not to hurt their feelings.

* * *

Then in the late eighties, Operation Rescue truly desegregated Catholic and Protestant pro-lifers in the best sense. We were together, taking non-violent action by blockading abortion facilities to save unborn babies. We were singing the same religious hymns from literally the same hymnal, praying aloud together, lying on the ground next to each other and being dragged away by police to jail together. It was scary, exhilarating and effective. And it was very ecumenical. From my small town there were three regular Rescuers, two Baptists and one Catholic—me. Bob Chernisky and I would get up on certain, prearranged Saturday mornings, the usual Operation Rescue day and meet at 4:30 a.m. As we would drive together, we sometimes would get into heavy conversations about our God and our differing faiths. We would go to a secretly pre-arranged New England meeting site near an abortion "clinic," park and join the other Christian Rescuers. We would then walk en masse to the surprised abortion site and lay down on the ground in front of the door to block the "clinic" entrance, so no abortions could be done. Hours later in handcuffs, we would be carried away, supine by police because we would not comply willingly to leave the site of baby killings. We saved Protestant, Catholic, Jewish, Buddhist, atheist and Muslim babies. Very ecumenical baby-saving!

"The Rescue Chronicles," a book by Attorney John Broderick of Long Island, New York relates historical anecdotes of the eighties and nineties Operation Rescue saga. One such anecdote describes a group of Rescuers, both Protestants and Catholics, imprisoned in a Vermont jail after a Rescue in Burlington. The prison administration decided, after many requests, to allow religious services for the Rescuers, but only for the Protestants. Catholics were denied the right to have Mass. The Protestants protested this injustice vociferously and were threatened with extra punishment by the jailers for their complaining. The Protestant Rescuers were so determined and forceful that they were successful and Catholics were allowed their own service also. That's true ecumenism and brotherly love.

Although I have been heavily influenced by the direct action and the baby-saving successes of Operation Rescue's blockades of the eighties and nineties, I realize that civil disobedience doesn't work anymore for pro-lifers. The court penalties are extreme and more severe than for any other type of civil disobedience. A rapist gets more rights than a 75 year old grandmother arrested in front of an abortion facility. The CPC Plus effort is strictly within the law and disadvantages only the abortion "clinics" not the civil authorities. Direct action can be lawful.

Catholic and Evangelical CPCs

Although the original Operation Rescue is long gone, that joint experience helped bring Christians of all faiths together. There are still real differences, however. For instance, from my experience, it is mostly Catholics that you see praying or sidewalk counseling in front of abortion mills although there are pockets of Evangelical sidewalk counseling efforts nationally. Evangelicals operate many of the small crisis pregnancy centers, usually distant from abortion mills, while Catholics tend to locate their CPCs near abortions "clinics." As I have previously written, Evangelical-run, crisis pregnancy centers seemed to be more interested in saving the soul of the pregnant woman, rather than saving her baby from abortion. Saving the baby is paramount in Catholic run centers. Catholics seem to get around to trying to reorder the woman's life, which could include God and church, after the baby is safe.

Volunteering within Churches

Many CPCs began as a mission from an Evangelical church or as Catholic laity trying to save babies. Some started with more than one church supporting it and providing volunteers. Because of these special beginnings, much of the personality and policy was brought over to the CPC. Faith, hope, peace and charity pervade the pro-life movement, unlike the so-called pro-choice movement with its millions of violent abortions. That depravity reaps only darkness, hatred, loneliness, despair, rage, ruin and decay. The organized pro-life groups within the movement have always condemned violence. There has never been a case of violence, toward an abortion intent woman by a pro-life activist. *Our movement is the largest public campaign in American history and the most peaceful.* Much of that can be attributed to our church influences. Those of us who are Christians can never get far from our God and His church.

For many years in my volunteer work, I have heard many of my Catholic fellow workers complain about the Catholic hierarchy. "Why doesn't the bishop do something about that (fill in the blank)?" It could be some scandalous Catholic politician or a new abortion facility. My answer has always been that we should not expect bishops or priests (or ministers, rabbis) to be political. They are not trained to be politicians. The clergy is trained to preach, to manage our parishes, to evangelize, and to bring Christ to us in the Eucharist and otherwise.

Some of us laypeople do not like politics but we must participate anyway. Pope Benedict XVI said the following, "The immediate task of action in the political field, to build a just order in society, does not correspond to the Church as such, but to the lay faithful, who act as citizens on their own responsibility." The laity must confront our sick society. We, lay people must call the politicians to task for their immoral votes. We, lay people must save babies, protest and pray on the streets in front of abortion mills, city halls and legislatures. We, lay people must actively work against the current, cultural spiral into decadence.

There is blame enough to go around for all Christians not just clergy. How did we let abortion grow so much that it is now so difficult to eliminate? Although Catholic bishops were early heroes, many of them became political ostriches, as Catholic politicians became the front row leaders in the expansion of abortion. Such politicians like Speaker Nancy Pelosi and Senator John Kerry even today, continue to receive Communion on Sunday and vote to kill babies on Tuesday. Our Church and our bishops can't let that continue!

Before Vatican II, RC lay people wanting to volunteer were restricted to Catholic Church authorized agencies that were run mostly within parishes and managed by the Church hierarchy. In other words at that time, those of us wanting to help poor people were restricted to volunteering at our parish's St. Vincent de Paul Society under the strong hand of the pastor. I think that one purpose of that crabbed system was to insure that agencies acting within the Church were faithful to its doctrines. The Church did not want Catholics working on projects whose goals were at cross-purposes to the Church's goals and doctrines. England's Cardinal John Henry Newman was a revolutionary in his time, suggesting that the laity could be used more effectively. Today Catholics volunteer without concern for that bureaucratic notion of hierarchical management. It is obvious that today some organizations for which Roman Catholics volunteer do operate at cross-purposes to the Church; e.g. Voice of the Faithful, Catholics for Free Choice, Catholic Health Association, etc.

Churches are a rich fountain of wonderful, talented and generous people. CPCs are very lucky to have any and all churches as benefactors.

12.

Who is the Enemy?

Since we are fighting against the horror of abortion, spending our valuable time and our treasure in this battle, we need to know against whom we are fighting. We need to know who are the enemies of human life. They are legion; abortionists, feminists, most lesbians and many male homosexuals, many academics, most Unitarians, many mainline Protestant churches, too many media people, the official Democrat Party, the country club Republicans, most Jewish activists but usually not Orthodox Jews and others. NARAL (National Abortion and Reproductive Rights Action League), NOW, National Abortion Federation (the abortionists' trade association), the Feminist Majority, and Planned Parenthood are some of the enemy's organizations.

Regarding the Democratic Party, if the pre-born had voting rights, there would be immediate legislation by Speaker Nancy Pelosi, et al to set up voter registration booths in all the abortionists' buffer zones in the U.S.A.

In 2006, Brian Clowes of Human Life International, did a thorough study, searching through 15 thousand IRS 990's (non-profit organization's annual filing forms) to see how balanced the funding was between pro-abortion and pro-life non-profits organizations. Pro-life groups raised $551 million in 2006 and pro-abortion groups raised $9.2 billion the same year. That figures out to 95 percent of the money going to pro-aborts and 5 percent going to pro-lifers. $461 million of the $551 million pro-life dollars went to crisis pregnancy centers, which is spending our small portion well, I think. Now we know why the battle is taking so long to win. But we will finally win, because God has guaranteed it.

Planned Parenthood alone took more than twice the take of every pro-life group in America in 2006. Planned Parenthood (PP) is the largest purveyor of abortion in the U.S.A. and probably the world. Lately the abortion rate has had a slight downtick, thanks be to God, but PP's rate has gone up. It seems that the independent abortionists can't compete with PP's political clout and lobbying ability to get government grants. As small abortionists (Should I call them mom and pop baby-killers?) thankfully go out of business, Planned Parenthood takes that "business" and its death rate and its sales numbers rise.

Pro-abortion groups often put out false news releases about how well funded pro-life pregnancy centers are. It is ludicrous when you know that Planned Parenthood's funding alone is twice what all the pro-life groups together receive in donations.

The U.S.A. Government Accountability Office (GAO) reported in 2010 that between 2002 and 2009 US taxpayers have paid one billion dollars to abortion advocacy groups: The Advocates for Youth—$8.7 million; Guttmacher Institute—$12.7 million; International Planned Parenthood - $93.8 million; Planned Parenthood Federation of America—$657.1 million; Population Council—$284.3 million and Sexuality Information and Education Council—$1.6 million.

Another example of this dishonesty is "Feministing," a pro-abort blog that recently ran the following breathless story, entitled, "Millions in federal funds go to crisis pregnancy centers." Their story reports that pro-abortion Congressman Henry Waxman complained that $30 million of federal funding for abstinence-only programs were funneled into what he calls anti-choice crisis pregnancy centers since 2001. The blog continues, "we can't forget that it's still millions of federal dollars being put into illegal and extremely harmful practices that are conducted in these supposedly 'safe spaces' for women to go when in need. . ." Any kind of aid the CPCs receive will bring out this kind of hysteria and hate.The enemy never rests.

* * *

STOPP (Stop Planned Parenthood), located in Stafford, Virginia, is completely focused on putting PP out of business.

If you have a Planned Parenthood in your area, STOPP has a plan to eliminate it. They are very creative with their ideas. Their website address is www.stopp.org.

They say that, if three people dedicate all their time beyond their working and family lives, working to shut down a specific Planned Parenthood facility, it could be done in three years. Whether it's been there for many years, or it just opened up makes no difference according to Jim Sedlak, STOPP Director. Maybe you have been fighting its coming and despite your best efforts, it has arrived. There are a number of legal, non-violent actions you can take to lessen Planned Parenthood's business and make it think about leaving. I would love such a three-person team to plague Planned Parenthood in Worcester, Massachusetts. Below is STOPP's battle plan.

Education—the first thing you should do is start educating your community.

Picketing—The single most effective thing you can do to fight an existing Planned Parenthood facility is to establish a regular (at least weekly) picket. This single act will lower PP's business, tarnish its community image, and result in increased public attention to its programs and philosophies. All these effects will work to your benefit. The more frequently you can picket PP's offices, the better. However, you should at least plan a weekly, two-hour picket. When you picket weekly, you do not need large numbers. The frequency will have its effect and will cause morale and business problems for PP. Most Planned Parenthood facilities do not perform surgical abortions (all provide the Pill, Depo Provera, and Emergency Contraception and, therefore, are providing the means for chemical abortions). If your PP does not do surgical abortions, your pickets should concentrate on chemical abortions (also called medical abortions). Primarily target the Pill and the fact that PP comes between local parents and their children.

Access to kids—Planned Parenthood is anxious to get to teens and younger children. It often establishes programs in schools and with the YWCA, Girl Scouts, Big Brothers, Big Sisters and anywhere else that kids, especially teens and pre-teens, gather. You should investigate each of these organizations in your town and if you find PP involved, get it out. You can educate the public to lessen PP's influence and get it "uninvited" to the groups

Access to money—Planned Parenthood needs money to operate and is very good at getting money from the various government agencies. You should investigate your local city, town and county governments and determine if any money is going to Planned Parenthood. If so, make a stink about it. In September 2010 Governor Chris Christie of New Jersey, because of severe budget restraints, defunded Planned Parenthood. Almost immediately the abortion organization started closing offices.

Newsletters—Once you start fighting against an already established Planned Parenthood facility, you should send a monthly newsletter to your supporters and all who sign your petitions. The newsletter need not be fancy but it should keep your people informed about what is happening. It can be used to notify them of weekly and special pickets, tell them of upcoming critical dates, and relate any successes you have experienced. In addition, you can include some national information on PP from STOPP International's Ryan Report. Our enemies are strong but Christ is much stronger and we have Him on our side.

Nasty NARAL

NARAL is stepping up its attacks against our pregnancy centers. In 2010 they have used their tame legislators and other henpecked political leaders in New York City, Austin, Texas; Baltimore and Montgomery County, Maryland to threaten and/or successfully impose wholly unjustified regulations requiring the posting of signs stating that the pro-life pregnancy centers do not provide or refer for abortions. Those regulations also require the centers to state on their signs, that they do not provide birth control services.

The latter claim is untrue because our centers do provide education about abstinence and natural family planning. This kind of unconstitutional harassment of pro-life centers will continue in other jurisdictions. Watch for it!

Why is NARAL so furiously against our current, faint-hearted, baby-saving efforts? I think they perceive a threat to the default abortion position, which currently prevails. Unplanned pregnancy = abortion is often the default position in America today. With the help of God, our centers and sidewalk counselors (especially it seems in New York, Maryland and Texas) continue to change thousands of women each week from abortion to life. That means fewer abortions and less income for the abortionists. That translates to less funding for NARAL since most of their funding comes from abortionists. Pregnancy centers threaten the dominance of NARAL, NOW (National Organization of Women), Planned Parenthood and the other abortionists. A better reason to start a CPC you couldn't find!

That pro-abortion hate and fury is highlighted by the remarks of Dr. Leroy Carhart, an active late term abortionist and a developer of the partial birth abortion technique. He is quoted at a July 2010 NOW conference in Boston, as saying, regarding pro-lifers, "Treat them like terrorists." At the same event NOW President Terry O'Neill added, "Unlimited detention. Freeze their assets." Beware of these hate filled people and pray for their conversion.

* * *

The Massachusetts Registry of Motor Vehicles finally approved a pro-life license plate in 2010 after a long and difficult effort by one pro-life woman – Merry Nordeen. I've got my beautiful plates on my pickup. NARAL was horrified that an image of a loving mother cradling an infant would be allowed on our state's auto plates. The legend bothers them too–"Choose Life." The Worcester Telegram newspaper published my letter to the editor soon after NARAL's public condemnation of this plate. I wrote, "If NARAL gets its own plate, then I suggest two legends"; "Choose Death" or "NARAL, Giving Life a Bad Name."

* * *

CPCs in general are seen by some college women in a hostile way. We must remember that pregnancy resource centers have enemies, who would like to shut us down. It seems strange that those who have appropriated the name "pro-choice" would want to make sure that a pregnant woman has no other choice but abortion. We must be aware and vigilant of pro-abortion fake clients and spies. NARAL's CPC Campaign was set up to investigate and record what it erroneously thinks are deceptive practices by pro-life pregnancy centers. Everything pregnancy centers do is honest, legal, and done with the best of intentions. Problem Pregnancy gets phony client calls and visits every year about the same time, at the beginning of the fall semester of Clark University's "Women's Studies" course. Instructors for that "course" are inevitably hard-core feminists.

Employing NARAL's dirty tricks, one or more of her students will call for an appointment, using a written script which we usually detect immediately. Our veteran counselors will tell her that when she arrives we will first need to check to see if she is pregnant. The pregnancy kit that tests a client's urine sample at our office is provided free. The fake clients, knowing they are not pregnant, usually give up at that point because their negative test result would kill the hoped-for counseling session. Most of them would have planned to bring in a hidden audio recorder or camera to record what they have been erroneously told is nefarious counseling. Some attempts have been made by fraudulent, non-pregnant clients to bring in a real pregnant woman's urine to fake the pregnancy test. We are aware of such gimmicks and foil them. These pretend clients will be nervous and avoid eye contact. Some will seem to know too much about what we pregnancy centers do. These young stooges almost always use fictitious names. NARAL provides a set script to follow at the CPC.

One of their games is that the fake client arrives with a different race boyfriend (e.g., black woman with white boyfriend), expecting to find and record racism from our counselors. Of course, what they do not know is that a majority of Problem Pregnancy's clients are either Latina or black. We have zero bias towards any client. Another trick is for a student to pose as if she is doing a research project on abortion. As a rule, we do not allow any student interviews of our counselors, even shutting out legitimate students. It is too risky because our enemies will invent wholly false and harmful conversations and try to publicize that fraud to hurt our reputation. During our beautiful New England autumn, we can expect stunning red, green and gold leaves to decorate the landscape and sunny but cool, brisk days but also we can expect fraudulent clients, profane graffiti and sometimes broken windows on our building, all inspired by the same feminist instructor or NARAL.

And the latest hissy fit, in the summer of 2010, NARAL started demanding that internet Yellow Page sites spike *all* CPC listings.

In August of 2010, Obama's FBI co-sponsored a "training session" with Planned Parenthood and its allies in Portland Oregon. The purpose was to declare the free speech of pro-life Americans as "violent". A spokesman for the pro-life Alliance Defense Fund responded, "The information presented in the seminar raises serious concerns over the . . . government's treatment of nonviolent free speech activities as 'violence' subject to investigation and prosecution," In the document derived from that meeting, there were about 140 purported incidents at American abortion facilities listed under Arson & Bombings, almost all phony or exaggerated. I am pleased Planned Parenthood in Worcester claimed one so-called incident (1990). Worcester pro-lifers would have felt left out otherwise. The pro-abortion vitriol continues to flow unabated.

13.

The Related Problem of Single Mothers Pregnant Again

Those of us who counsel women regarding abortion have seen countless women for whom chaos is a way of life. Many of those women become mothers without husbands, raising children without fathers. I am very sympathetic to those women. The fathers of their babies are of the masculine gender but in my opinion are not real men or as our Jewish brethren would say, "They are not mensch."

Irresponsibility has become an epidemic among young American men. 40 percent of American children go to sleep in a home, where no father lives. Too often though, a series of the mothers' boyfriends *are* sleeping there. Surveys of American children consistently show that kids without fathers and/or kids from broken families are much more likely to drop out of school, take drugs, get into trouble with the police and earn less money in their lifetimes than kids from intact families. Of course, this is not the only determinant. According to the U.S. Census Bureau, there are 10 million single mothers in the U.S.A. That adds up to at least 10 million kids without fathers, and likely more. Finances are almost always the biggest concern for these mothers. Day-care, costing $5 thousand a year or more is another big problem. Hopelessness and despair are the single mother's most constant companions.

Many single mothers were abandoned by the men who got them pregnant. They are bitter because they are with children but without marriage and without a husband. One of the strongest needs for these women is to deal with the resentment, the anger, and the outrage felt for the men, who took advantage of them. Often the woman was convinced that she was loved and that the man was committed to her. She was conned and gave up probably the only thing she had of value – her body and sex. Too often she was abandoned immediately after becoming pregnant. The result for the woman, besides having to raise the children by herself, is lots of anger, resentment, and ambivalence about men.

Although it seems easy to say for this writer, a man, who has had an intact family from his earliest days up to today, it is still a fact that single mothers need to pray to God, the Father to be the Father of the fatherless. She should teach her kids to ask for strength and wisdom, to allow Christ, the Son, to guide her and them. The whole family should pray to the Holy Spirit for wisdom, courage and peace. The three Persons of the Holy Trinity are the answer for all of us, no matter how tough our life is.

Additional support systems to help single mothers and their children are needed. I have read statistics citing that two thirds of all single mothers have not completed high school and that we add 465,000 teen single mothers every year. The bible (James 1:27) says that we should care for widows and orphans. Pro-lifers, neighbors and other people should search out opportunities to help single mothers. Look for ways to aid her without embarrassing her. Today's single mothers and their fatherless children qualify as widows and orphans as far as I am concerned. A woman's extended family is the logical source of support for her but often that is missing.

Such women need good advice on raising children from those who have done it well like us. One thing a single mother should be very concerned about is adult male predators. These men are the lowest form of human life. We sometimes see them at Problem Pregnancy with their girlfriends, now pregnant. Some of them actually take pride in serially fathering babies, one naïve young woman after another, one orphan after another. They prey on single mothers with low self-esteem and a small income, often welfare only. They move in to the woman's apartment or just become overnight guests. Their pretence of love for the women turns into "borrowing" or stealing the children's welfare money. Sometimes these men prey sexually on her children also. We read stories of these guys, being arrested for horrendous physical abuse, rape and even the murder of the unprotected children, while supposedly babysitting these vulnerable kids.

We live in a predatory society, and single mothers can't afford to ignore this. They should be careful about the people counted on for childcare. Family members usually make the best providers. Unless the mother knows the other adults living in the home of the caregiver she should never leave her children there.

How does a single mother pass on to her son male attributes like masculine honor, pride and that mysterious thing nicknamed "macho"? Peggy Drexler ("Raising Boys without Men") argues that it is only poverty and not father absence that hurts children. She is wrong! She says boys are hardwired to grow into men. Yes, but they are not hardwired to grow into good responsible, family men. That is a job for mothers and fathers working together.

14.

Little Things We Can Do

Many of my readers may not be able to jump right in to the CPC Plus project, because of family or job responsibilities. Maybe they would still like to do something to stop abortion. Below is a list of suggestions.

The point of this list is to offset the negative zeitgeist prevailing in our culture today regarding motherhood, fatherhood, pregnancy, big families and the healthy discipline of our children. Our popular culture provides examples like "the lovable rogue" father who never advances beyond his irresponsible adolescence. And don't forget the People Magazine-ization of our time with its fourth-grade level, relativist philosophy of "live and let live." Additionally our movies and media bring us also what has always been a masculine fault but is intensifying - the objectification of a woman's body parts, excusive of the woman herself.

I had started to list some of these offsetting good ideas, when I read a Mary Meehan column that listed much better suggestions to help the pro-life movement. I have amalgamated Meehan's list into my own.

Tell a mother how beautiful her baby is.

Tell pregnant mothers how happy you are for them and ask if they need help.

Tell pregnant mothers how pregnancy makes a woman so healthy and so beautiful. I think women glow when they are pregnant.

Financially support crisis pregnancy centers. Check the yellow pages under "Abortion Alternatives" for the ones nearest you.

Encourage adoption. Read about it and defend the concept when others are criticizing it.

If you are a doctor or medical student, talk with colleagues about the way abortion adversely affects your profession. Offer your services free to pregnant mothers in need.

If you are a lawyer or law student, question the pro-abortion concepts that have crept into the legal profession. Look for pro-bono legal work that will foster the Culture of Life.

Many facets of the pro-life movement are woefully under-covered by the media. If you are a writer or reporter, there is a real need for serious investigative reporting on the lack of abortion clinic data, the amount of money earned in this "business," etc.

Men should talk to other men, especially to young men, about male responsibility regarding women, pregnancy and children.

Be complimentary to mothers and fathers raising large families. Tell them how wonderful that is. Offer help if it seems to be needed.

Discourage jokes about abortion or Christian efforts against abortion.

Support educational efforts to discourage abortion. Financially support pro-life sources of books, magazines, articles, television and radio programs.

Keep an eye on your elected officials. Vote them out if they are pro-abortion.

Raise your boys to be responsible men and good fathers.

Raise your girls to demand that their boyfriends and potential husbands be first judged as good father material.

Pray!

15.

Life on the Abortion Frontline

Below are a few anecdotes from almost thirty years of fighting abortion and saving babies in Worcester. Some are from my notes and from previous Problem Pregnancy appeal letters and some were given to me by sidewalk counselors.

Tap on the Window Babies

Our sidewalk counselors, who must work around an unjust buffer zone, get few good opportunities to speak to clients as they drive quickly by us into the fenced Planned Parenthood parking area. The Worcester abortionist has strategically located 360-degree cameras monitored by a security guard who constantly watches the two Planned Parenthood entrances.

When our sidewalk counselors get the chance to speak to a potential turnaround, we take it and quickly. Nancy C., one of our most successful sidewalk counselors told me that sometimes a client's car will stop halfway into the abortionist parking lot. Nancy will immediately go the woman's side of the car and "tap on the window." Sometimes the client will open the window and counseling begins. Nancy calls those babies she saves in this manner, "Tap on the Window" babies.

Holiday Baby-Saving

There are times in Worcester when the security guard doesn't want to come out to enforce the buffer zone. It might a brutal, sweltering 100-degree day or a frigid, five-degree January day or maybe he is hung-over or just lazy. Our sidewalk counselors take full advantage of those opportunities by going into the verboten parking lot to speak to the clients. Usually that opportunity will close after a short time but we often can save a baby when it happens. When the abortionist office closes on what is ordinarily a usually scheduled abortion days such as around a holiday, an opportunity to save babies becomes available. Some clients, not realizing that the "clinic" is closed, will show up without appointments and drive into the parking lot. But the closure allows us to go right into the fenced parking lot to speak to the woman. The buffer zone only applies when the abortionist is open. Because Problem Pregnancy may be closed also, this baby-saving gambit requires a trained counselor who could handle inside counseling along with sidewalk counseling.

Some Recent Baby-Saves

Recently our counselor Kathy L. saw a client who had more than the usual personal, financial and medical problems including one of her five children being mentally ill. After Kathy tried everything to persuade the client not to abort, the woman left and the prognosis was that the baby was a goner. Then two weeks later the woman came in to the office again. She told Kathy that she thought about all of our counseling and particularly about our offer of substantial aid if the baby were allowed to live. The client agreed to "keep" the baby, if we could help her with two big problems. One was that we pay an overdue and overwhelming, $13 hundred heating bill and the other was that we pay for repairs to get her junker car back on the road. We said yes to both and the baby will live.

Jean W., another great counselor told me about a couple who came to us thinking that we were Planned Parenthood. During the first session Jean thought the father/husband did not want an abortion but that the mother did. They left without a resolution but with an ultrasound appointment for the following week. On the day of the ultrasound, Jean looked out into our parking lot and saw the husband trying to get his wife out of their car. The wife was crying and fighting to stay in the car and the husband was pulling her and threatening her. Jean ran out and soon figured out that it was the wife who did not want an abortion. The husband/father was abortion instigator. Neither spouse realized that we were not abortionists and that they were not at Planned Parenthood. It took Jean 20 minutes of pleading to finally get the wife to understand that we would not kill her baby. She finally left her car and Jean worked with her. She is being helped with practical things and the baby will live. When he discovered that no abortion would happen, the husband stormed out of our office and left his pregnant wife.

Some Older Baby-Saving Anecdotes

A few years ago Sharon (pseudonym), originally abortion-intent but changed by our ultrasound scan, came to us with James, her newborn for diapers and formula. It was a very busy day and our great counselors, Helen and Chris, were dealing with many other clients so Sharon and baby James were in the office waiting area. Another abortion-intent client, Bonita (pseudonym) was sitting near Sharon in the waiting area and the two women began to talk. Sharon discovered that Bonita had an abortion appointment next door at Planned Parenthood. Somehow Bonita had arrived mistakenly at our pro-life center, thanks be to God. Both Bonita and Sharon had very similar situations – single, irresponsible boyfriends, etc. Counselor Helen, overwhelmed with clients and seeing Sharon begin to try to convince Bonita against aborting her child, sent them (with baby James) into a counseling room alone and shut the door. This was a first for us and an inspired idea because 30 minutes later Bonita came out turned around and wanting to deliver her baby. The two women had become fast friends, exchanging phone numbers and promising to help one another through coming difficult times.

* * *

Anya (pseudonym) was in the abortion facility next door being prepared for an abortion when a Planned Parenthood staffer mistakenly allowed a corner of the ultrasound screen to be seen by Anya. (Abortionists but not clients are allowed to see the babies on ultrasound at Planned Parenthood. When the client saw her baby moving on the screen, she panicked, jumped off the table and ran out of the building where our outside counselor steered her to our office. We counseled her and showed her a full ultrasound screen of her baby and she wept with relief. Anya kept crying and saying, "I almost killed my baby. I almost killed my baby." One saved baby!

Marilee (pseudonym) called a few years ago on our hotline and spoke to Sheila, one of our great hotline counselors and told her a long but happy-ending story, which I have shortened. Marilee was one of our first ultrasound clients. She later called to tell us how grateful she was that we were there to show her what she carried in her womb. She said that she was determined to have an abortion but once she saw her baby on the screen, she couldn't do it. Her new baby was born that spring and Marilee was bubbling over with joy and gratitude. Another saved baby!

Lena (pseudonym) was sitting in Planned Parenthood's waiting room with an abortion appointment. She was still not 100 percent sure about her "choice." She later told us that she was depressed by the desperate atmosphere in the abortion facility's waiting room. She said the other waiting clients seemed so very sad and many were crying. She had previously seen our sign and then like Anya she "escaped" and came over to Problem Pregnancy "to talk about it." We counseled her and showed her baby on the ultrasound screen. Lena told us, as many others do every week, "I couldn't kill my baby after seeing her on the screen." And another saved baby! Results of 3 cases = 3 Saved Babies and 3 Happy Mothers!

Three Miracles at Problem Pregnancy

We, Problem Pregnancy volunteers have become rather blasé about God's miracles that regularly happen (for 28 years) at our baby-saving center. But I'm often asked by our supporters for reports of some of these miracle stories. I think a larger audience would appreciate them too. So here are three.

In July (2004) Kon (pseudonym), a Korean immigrant client came to our office with a 4 month old, beautiful baby boy and an amazing story of how perilous is the life of an unborn baby today since abortion became legal up to the last day of pregnancy. It began the previous November when Kon came to us, unmarried and pregnant by another Asian immigrant. Both demanded an abortion. Even after counseling, they were still adamant for the abortion. Kon told us that she was concerned for her own health because of debilitating Lupus. They did agree to an ultrasound and thereby discovered a baby boy. Immediately the father decided he wanted the baby boy. If the scan had shown a girl, she would be dead. Kon, outwardly acquiescent to her man. agreed to life for the baby. As usual, Kon received a set of scan photos in a little colorful baby album. Kon's baby's due date was March 2004.

But now "the rest of the story." This proud Momma with beautiful son confessed to us that at 25 weeks pregnant, she again changed her mind and decided to have an abortion after all. She then checked all the abortionists in Massachusetts and none would do such a late term abortion. So Kon and her sister drove 1600 miles from Worcester to Wichita, Kansas to the notorious Dr. George Tiller's late term abortuary (now closed). Incredibly, the late Dr. Tiller killed babies right up to the delivery date. His nickname among pro-lifers was "Tiller the Killer." She was still carrying her PPW ultra-sound photos when she arrived in Wichita. Kon then had another change of heart in her Kansas hotel room after looking again at the ultrasound photo album and so the two drove back another 1600 miles to Worcester. In March she delivered a healthy baby.

So our ultrasound actually saved that little boy twice, once because the scan showed he had the father-required male plumbing and the second time when the mother looked again at the ultrasound photos in Kansas. By the grace of God the baby is very much loved by both parents and the mother came to thank us. By the way, a possible second miracle? – Kon is now completely Lupus free.

A $10,000 Miracle on the Roof—Miracle #2

In June 2003 Problem Pregnancy was able to buy the building we had been renting (625 Lincoln Street) next door to Planned Parenthood's abortion facility. It took every dollar we had plus a large bank mortgage. Many very generous supporters helped us with the down payment and we thank them again. Our mortgage payment was a little less than our rent payment was. In the past our abortionist neighbor, because of our aggressive baby-saving efforts, was able to get us evicted from other locations. No one can ever evict PPW again from our baby-saving location. But that was last year's miracle.

During the very rainy spring we discovered the "joys" of building ownership – our flat roof had developed very bad leaks and was ruining the ceilings, etc. After much prayer and research, we decided to not just repair the roof but to tear it off and replace it with a long-lasting, slanted rubber membrane roof. The shocking prices ranged from $33 thousand and up. Finally we were able to find a family of roofers, two of who were PPW supporters, who would do the job for $10 thousand in labor costs. Under this plan we would save by buying the materials wholesale ($10 thousand) bringing the total to $20 thousand that we didn't have. I prayed and began to "put the arm" on some of our supporters. Relatively quickly we raised $10 thousand and bought the materials.

This capital expense could not be stalled. Good weather was necessary for the roof installation and "mañana was not good enough" anymore. This roofing family was available weekends and nights only. We arranged for them to begin Memorial Day weekend. We prayed they would have the needed four days of good weather. I still didn't know where the remaining $10 thousand would come from. The materials were delivered. A huge dumpster was dropped off for the debris from the old roof. They began and the weather was excellent throughout the four days – no rain. These men worked from 6 a.m. to 11 p.m. noisily tearing up the roof, pounding, sawing, nailing, etc. The neighbors even called the police one late night about the din. On the fourth day most of the work was done but I was told that another weekend was needed to finish it up. Thankfully, that gave me another week to come up with the dough!

On Saturday morning of the following weekend, the job was almost finished and the money was to be paid within hours. There was a Mass in our chapel, celebrated by Fr. Michael Roy, while the pounding went on above. I prayed again as I had been praying, asking God to help us pay for the work. As I do on Saturdays after Mass. I went to check our post office box at the nearby post office. There were the usual bills, some address change returns, a few small donations, and mixed with some junk mail was a big gray, mysterious envelope. I opened it and was shocked. There was a $10 thousand anonymous donation to Problem Pregnancy in the form of a bank check with no evidence of who was the donor—*the exact amount needed for the laborers!*

When I went back to PPW, I was cheering and praising God and Fr. Roy was cheering with me. He and I agreed that God provides if something is needed for the right cause. *This time He provided the very roof over our mothers' and babies' heads.*

Carla (pseudonym) came to our office on a beautiful spring day but she did not feel very beautiful. She was unmarried, pregnant and wanted an abortion. She also had a history of depression and was possibly suicidal. She was in her twenties and described herself as a born-again Christian. Her life, however, was a mess. Joanne, one of our great lay counselors, showed her the fetal models, various pro-life videos and lovingly advised her. At the end of this agonizing session, Carla had changed her mind and decided not to have an abortion. As we do with all our clients, a small pro-life token is given when leaving. Carla was given a tiny, exact size pink, plastic, unborn baby replica. Our busy office then went on to other clients until a follow up call to Carla found that she had changed her mind back to abortion. Joanne again convinced her back to life for the baby. After that, our calls were never returned. We never knew the outcome and we worried about Carla and her little one.

One day a phone call came from a Boston psychiatric hospital. It was a pro-life nurse, probably breaking hospital rules, telling us that Carla was at her psychiatric ward. We were told that she had gone to a Boston abortionist and was signed in and waiting, when she was asked for the expected $5 hundred. She went into her purse, searching. As she pulled out the money, out popped the little pink, plastic baby. She had forgotten it and all the pro-life counseling she had suppressed came back in a torrent. It devastated her. She emotionally broke into pieces. She wept and couldn't go through with the abortion. Soon after, she ended up in that psychiatric ward. She is now healing and wants us to know how grateful she is for our little pink plastic baby. According to Carla, happily, it was the cause of her being unable to kill her own baby.

Afterword

The Equilibrium That Will Save Babies' Lives

Equilibrium is the condition of a system in which competing influences are balanced. If pro-lifers are really serious about fighting abortion, then we must rhetorically whip the anti-lifers with their own word – choice. When feminists use the word – choice—they mean an unbalanced system with only one option – abortion. We need to improve our offer to abortion minded women and then argue our case better. The pro-abortion folks' limiting of choices should become their biggest weakness. We need to take advantage of their sophistry. We need to take the argument to potential clients and to the public in every way possible. The argument that the word—choice—of course requires not one but two options. It's mathematical. One option is abortion. There must be another preference in order to complete that mathematical equation and to bring the needed balance to the pregnant mother. Pro-lifers must provide the *other option* to women. What is that other option? I think we announce from the rooftops that American pregnancy centers provide *real* and sometimes expensive, substantial aid where necessary to pregnant needy women.

Of course we would target a particular population of pregnant mothers. Those who would be receptive to our offer of needed substantial aid and quid pro quo, not abort their babies. This is the group we are failing. From a purely self-absorbed, un-churched pregnant mother's vantage point, most pregnancy centers and sidewalk counseling efforts do *not* provide truly practical alternatives for that desperate pregnant woman and thus often leave her with only the abortion choice. But if American pregnancy centers offered real, practical and often expensive help, then that woman would have equilibrium—a real choice. I'm including costly things, like paying an apartment's first, last and security deposit, paying for childcare or buying a car for the client. Real things that will change a mother's mind away from abortion. Until we do that, we do not truly offer another option to abortion for our target population of today's hardened, secularized, pregnant women. So to recapitulate, the options for that type of needy pregnant mother are the following:

Number 1 Choice.
Abortion. <u>Baby dies</u>.

Number 2 Choice.
Substantial help to the mother. <u>Baby lives</u>.

That equation will be a reality when the CPC Plus program or something like it goes national.

* * *

Why have I been able to start and operate CPC Plus agencies? I am not that smart. Successfully beginning such a baby-saving organization is not easy but the difficult parts should be done incrementally. Do not picture the whole process of starting the agency. Instead, pick out the smaller components, like incorporating a non-profit or finding an office very near an abortionist. Then afterwards do the other components, one by one. If there is no baby-saving effort at the location now, then anything is an improvement. Do what you can on the project as quickly as possible. That would be progress. Always move forward. Always pray for help but keep pushing forward. Voila! Before you know it, most of it will be done. That's the way I do everything. Keep copious notes for explaining everything to your board later. So get going!

At the end of the Appendix is a compiled list of the known abortion facilities in all 50 states. It is very thorough. I have tried unsuccessfully to find the origin of this list. I have added some abortionists to the original list. There are 12 abortion sites in my state. With this list, you can see where to set up your local CPC Plus and where to begin to compete for American babies' lives. Now that you have this book and this list, I issue a challenge – set up your center near your "favorite" abortionist and start saving babies' lives! Join me. You can do it!

Appendix

Three Examples of My Appeal Letters

1. The following is what I call my Super Letter. It had no graphics or photos, but it was powerful. I first used it in 1995 and it brought in more money at that time than any other previous appeal letter. I think it was a hit because it broadened the audience by suggesting that even pro-abortion people could support Problem Pregnancy. In our newer letters we have added a credit card payment option within the coupon at the end.

Pro-Life? Pro-Choice? Pro-Family?

What's all that mean? Where do I fit?

Dear friend,

No matter which of these designations you put on yourself, there still should be places for young, troubled, pregnant women without resources to get free help. Some results from the glaring inadequacy of such resources are:

* High infant death rates among minorities and the poor.
* Sickly, low weight babies caused by the lack of prenatal care.
* Young lonely, single mothers being preyed on, sexually and financially by older adult men. (Recent independent studies show that a large percentage of teenage pregnancies were fathered by destructive, irresponsible adults in their late twenties and thirties.)

* Rootless, young mothers abusing drugs, alcohol and sex and not taking care of their babies.
* Very high rates of venereal disease and AIDS in this young single mother population.
* Homeless young women living with their babies in whatever (often dangerous) places they can.
* 1.600,000 abortions every year in America.

Shouldn't there be a better way? At least in Central Massachusetts., there is! PROBLEM PREGNANCY OF WORCESTER, INC., a pro-life, volunteer agency, run by women, is a free, crisis pregnancy center. Our trained volunteer counselors provide **free**:

* **Housing and financial help.**
* **Medical referrals for prenatal health care.**
* **Prenatal nutrition.**
* **Adoption information.**
* **Maternity clothes; baby clothes; cribs; car seats; high chairs, etc.**
* **Down-to-earth counseling on STDs (sexually transmitted diseases).**

We have legal help available and everything is free. We are a complete aid center for the troubled women. Our motherly volunteers offer advice on (often lacking) life skills such as:

* **Alcohol and drug abuse reform; childcare and child nutrition.**
* **Home economics, home safety, medicine safety; miscarriages; SIDS.**
* **Getting free from abusive and parasitic boyfriends.**
* **Getting a GED and just generally getting chaotic lives back together.**

All this costs money! We are always under pressure financially. No one gets paid at PROBLEM PREGNANCY. Everyone is a volunteer. 100% of the donations go for care of women and children. We are nonsectarian, nonprofit and donations are deductible. We ask you whatever your pro or anti designation to help these unfortunate women and babies. Please send back the enclosed coupon and reply envelope and become a PP INC. supporter.

```
Rod Murphy, Director

Will you help?
$25___$50___$75___$100___$250___$500___$1000___$2000_
__Other___

Name_____

Address_____

City_____State____Zip_____Phone_

Send to Problem Pregnancy of Worcester, Inc.
```

* * *

2. This example was sent at Thanksgiving in 2006. I eliminated the graphics, the photos and the return coupon for this book. It is simple and was a great fundraiser.

Thanksgiving, 2006

Saving a Baby in the Language of Christ
Dear Supporter,

A few years ago I sent an appeal letter that addressed using foreign languages to save babies. Here's another one and it's a doozie! A women physician (XXXX) originally from an Arab country became a client at PPW. Ten years ago she had had an abortion and was suffering depression because of it. XXXX has become very pro-life and took one of our brochures used to sway women from abortion. She translated it to her native language – Aramaic, the language of Jesus. She posted it to an Aramaic website. Soon after XXXX received an email from another Mass. woman who had read her anti-abortion Aramaic brochure and decided not to abort her child. Do you think Jesus monitors familiar Aramaic websites and intervenes to help?

Even further XXXX came to PPW one day and volunteered to help us with clients especially Arabic or Aramaic speaking ones. At that precise time, we had an abortion minded client in the ultrasound room. XXX went in and spoke to the client, "Don't do it. I killed my baby 10 years ago and I deeply regret it". The two women then sat and talked and cried about their similar experiences. The client changed her mind and the baby lives because of that pro-life doctor.

What Does Problem Pregnancy Do and Why?

Recently I was challenged by a critic of our pro-life work. She asked, "So you manage to change the mind of a woman and she now has a new baby with almost no resources. What do you do to help her raise that newborn? What happens to that unwanted baby? Is it not better to abort that baby to avoid a miserable life?" Even among good people, I think, such a question might be asked.

Because of the almost complete lack of religious formation of young people today, most of us grow up with a utilitarian point of view toward life, as the critic exposed by her last question. If we analyze her questions, we should all be shocked. She is proposing that if a person cannot be assured of a life without trouble, poverty and hard knocks, etc., then someone should kill that person before birth (maybe later?). Also by her question, she is forecasting that every poor woman will deliver a baby that will be unwanted, poor and have a miserable life. But in the real world some rich kids, some middle class kids and some poor kids have miserable lives. But most people from each of those groups have good lives. Furthermore she solves the miserable-life problem by snuffing out the poor pre-born baby's life. Do you know of any person going through tough problems who would rather be euthanized? Our critic's position might better be called barbarism.

What's our solution? We are optimistic about mothers including mothers of surprise babies. Unwanted babies become loved and pampered even by poor families. Our mission is simple and definitive. We try to save babies on their way to being killed by abortion. We do it by helping a woman in any way we can to solve ancillary problems, so she doesn't want (or need) an abortion anymore. *We can not do everything!* We are a small volunteer outfit with limited resources. We do many things for our clients like becoming the loving aunt that a desperate woman needs and paying their rent, finding them housing, doctors and day care. We pay tuition, fix junky cars, provide diapers, baby food, cribs, car seats, and a hundred other things. We have our hands full right now. If a critic thinks there should be more comprehensive help after a client has her baby, we would be pleased to help that critic start another charity to do that job. We need your financial support to do our baby-saving job. We now take credit card donations. Please be generous

Thanks from the babies,

Rod Murphy, Director

* * *

3. This example was sent to supporters in 2008. It allows donors to see, how we have spent existing donors' money. Our supporters liked the openness. I removed the photos but left the return coupons.

SO HOW ARE WE DOING WITH YOUR MONEY?

For over 26 years we have asked you for financial gifts four times a year and you have generously responded. But do we deserve your donations? Does Problem Pregnancy save babies and help pregnant women? Are we good stewards of your money? Let's see how we're doing.

Babies Saved Two Ways

We have two levels within our organization to save babies from abortion—our intake counseling and our ultrasound test program. Our great women counselors turn around most of our pregnant clients from abortion during the initial counseling procedures (fetal models, films, offers of various aid, etc.). Planned Parenthood(unwillingly)and God provide us with many abortion-determined pregnant women. We are very effective with that population—saving maybe 80% but losing the other 20% of those babies as their hardened mothers go next door to the abortionist. And we have another level (and what a technological marvel) to offset that. See our *startling* ultrasound results.

80% Ultrasound Save Rate!

Since November '01 we have had an ultrasound program run by K.L., R.N. Those women participating are the toughest cases, not swayed by the above initial counseling. We

210

estimate turnarounds on <u>80%</u> of those most difficult situations! Some of these women have had previous abortions. Most were under extreme pressure from the baby's father or her family to "get rid of it". But seeing their own baby on the screen moving around and the gentle but tough-love approach of K.L. and L.M. (sonographers) persuade and allow maternal love and new life to prevail.

Youth Chastity Program

Our ultrasound is also being used to educate local teens before they need to make a "choice". Our Chastity/ Abstinence Outreach Program targets church schools, Catholic, Protestant and Orthodox. The youngsters with their teachers and clergy see a married pregnant mother being scanned by our ultrasound machine in real-time. LM and KL run these free classes at our pregnancy center. The kids are prepared at earlier church classes with an excellent Christian film about chastity. After the eye-popping view of a real baby moving in utero, those kids are shown a tough film about abortion. We don't hold back. The students' reactions are almost all positive with questions like this, "Why aren't we warned about this in school?" and "Do abortionists really do that to babies"?

Planting new CPCs and homes for mothers.

In 2006 we opened our first satellite office, Problem Pregnancy of North Quabbin in Athol. That North County area has a high teen pregnancy rate and Planned Parenthood targets that High school population with their pernicious and deadly propaganda. We are filling a needed abortion alternative in the area. We also believe that we have a responsibility to help others start pregnancy centers. So we have aided in the founding of at least three other free pregnancy centers in New England. Currently we are working on two more. Also Problem Pregnancy folks were instrumental in establishing Visitation House, the Worcester area home for pregnant women, who would otherwise be homeless because they won't "choose" abortion. We encourage such pro-life centers to offset the overwhelming pro-abortion cultural influences.

Providing a Worcester home for pro-life activities; meetings, etc.

Problem Pregnancy has always welcomed other pro-life and church groups that need a place to meet. Our office is constantly in use by other groups to further God's work in Central Mass. Because of our long successful history and our unshrinking advocacy for our pre-born, tiny brothers and sisters, we are the hub of pro-life activity in Central Mass. and beyond.

So are we deserving of your donation?

So for those who currently donate, do you now feel you are getting your money's worth? Did I mention that we are all volunteers and no one is paid? And for those yet to donate, if you want an effective pro-life organization that spends your money carefully yet saves real babies every week, Problem Pregnancy and our babies and mothers need your charity. Please help with a generous check.

Thanks from the babies,

Rod Murphy, Chairman

p.s. Problem Pregnancy has joined a national non-profit association (Leave a Legacy) that helps us in aiding any of our supporters who would like to name our organization (therefore our babies and mothers) as a beneficiary in their wills, etc. If you would like to know more, call our office and ask for Rod

Please be generous to our mothers and babies!
Or my check or cash in the amount
$25____$50____$75____$100____$250____$500____$1000___$2000 ____$5000____Other___

American Abortionists by City and State

ALABAMA - 7 Locations

New Woman All Women Health 1001 17th St. S. Birmingham, AL 35205

Planned Parenthood of Alabama 1211 27th Place S. Birmingham, AL 35205

Alabama Women's Center for Reproductive Alternatives 612 Madison St. SE Huntsville, AL 35801

Planned Parenthood 717 Downtowner Loop West Mobile, AL 36609

Beacon Women's Center 1011 Monticello Ct. Montgomery, AL 36117

Reproductive Health Services of Montgomery 811 South Perry St. Montgomery, AL 36109

West Alabama Women's Center 535 Jack Warner Pkwy. NE, # I Tuscaloosa, AL 35404

ALASKA - 5 Locations

Alaska Women's Health Services 4115 Lake Otis Pkwy. Anchorage, AK 99508

Planned Parenthood 4001 Lake Otis Parkway Anchorage, AK 99508

Planned Parenthood 1867 Airport Way, Ste. 160B Fairbanks, AK 99701

Planned Parenthood 3231 Glacier Hwy. Juneau, AK 99801

Dr. Michael Merrick 416 Frontage Rd., Ste. 400 Kenai, AK 99611

ARIZONA - 9 Locations

Abortion Services of Phoenix 3549 E. Cambridge Ave. Phoenix, AZ 85008

Acacia Women's Center 1615 E Osborn Rd Ste 100 Phoenix, AZ 85016

Camelback Family Planning 4141 N. 32nd Street, #105 Phoenix, AZ 85018

Family Planning Assoc. Med. Grp. 1331 N. 7th St., # 225 Phoenix, AZ 85006

Planned Parenthood 4417 N. 7th Ave. Phoenix, AZ 85013

Woman's Choice 5040 N. 15th Ave., # 204A Phoenix, AZ 85015

Planned Parenthood 1250 E. Apache Blvd., # 108 Tempe, AZ 85281

Old Pueblo Family Planning 5240 E. Knight Dr., # 112 Tucson, AZ 85712

Planned Parenthood 2255 N. Wyatt Rd. Tucson, AZ 85712

ARKANSAS - 2 Locations

Fayetteville Women's Clinic Dr. William Harrison 1011 N College Ave Fayetteville, AR 72701

Little Rock Family Planning Services 4 Office Park Dr. Little Rock, AR 72211

CALIFORNIA – 114 Locations

Family Planning Assoc. Med. Grp. 2500 H Street, Ste.100 Bakersfield, CA 93301

Brandeis Medical Center 8420 Wilshire Blvd. #27 Beverly Hills, CA 90211

Her Smart Choice/Clinica Los Remedios Dr. Vikram Kothandaraman 50 N Cienega Blvd. Ste. 218 Beverly Hills, CA 90211

Planned Parenthood 556 Vallombrosa Ave. Chico, CA 95926

Dr. Feliciano Rios 1079 3rd Ave Ste.C Chula Vista, CA 91911

Women's Health Specialists 1469 Humboldt Rd., # 200 Chico, CA 95928

A Woman's Choice 1550 Broadway Chula Vista, CA 91911

Dr. Fred Schnepper 765 Medical Center Ct. Ste. 209 Chula Vista, CA 91913

Choice Medical Group 2385 High School Ave. Concord, CA 94520

Planned Parenthood 2185 Pacheco St. Concord, CA 94520

Family Planning Assoc. Med. Grp. 8635 Firestone Blvd., # 100 Downey, CA 90241

Dr. Neysa Whiteman 477 N. El Camino Real Ste C-302 Encinitas, CA 92024

Center for Comprehensive Womens Health 5525 Etiwanda Ave # 216 Encino, CA 91356

Dr. Ying Chen 735 E. Ohio Ave Ste. 201 Escondido, CA 92025

Planned Parenthood 3225 Timer Fall Ct. Eureka, CA 95503

Planned Parenthood 1325 Travis Blvd., # C Fairfield, CA 94533

Women's Health Center 850 Sequoia Circle Fort Bragg, CA 95437

Choice Medical Group Fremont 1895 Mowry Avenue, Suite 116 Fremont, CA 94538

Family Planning Assoc. Med. Grp. 165 N. Clark St. Fresno, CA 93701

Planned Parenthood 650 North Fulton Fresno, CA 93728

Family Planning Assoc. Med. Grp. 372 Arden Ave., # 200 Glendale, CA 91203

A Pro-Choice Clinic 1290 B St., # 305 Hayward, CA 94541

Planned Parenthood 1866 B Street Hayward, CA 94541

Family Planning Medical Clinic 1840 N Hacienda Blvd Ste #13 La Puente, CA 91744

Planned Parenthood 14623 Hawthorne Blvd., # 300 Lawndale, CA 90260

Family Planning Assoc. Med. Grp., Dr. Robert Santella, Dr. Soon C. Sohn 2777

Long Beach Blvd., # 200 Long Beach, CA 90806

Alternatives Family Planning 3756 Santa Rosalia Dr., # 212 Los Angeles, CA 90008

Butterfly Medical Clinic 3756 Santa Rosalia Dr Suite # 220 Los Angeles, CA 90008

Clinica Medica Femenia 2010 Wilshire Blvd., # 610 Los Angeles, CA 90057

Family Planning Assoc. Med. Grp. 601 S. Westmoreland Ave. Los Angeles, CA 90005

Her Medical Clinic 2502 Figueroa St. #54 Los Angeles, CA 90007

Her Smart Choice/Clinica Los Remedios Dr. Vikram Kothandaraman 2226 E Cesar E Chavez Ave. Los Angeles, CA 90033

Her Smart Choice/Clinica Los Remedios Dr. Vikram Kothandaraman 2400 W. 7th St. Ste. 114 Los Angeles, CA 90057

La Costa Family Planning 2010 Wilshire Blvd., #55 Los Angeles, CA 90057

Pacific Women's Health Care 11101 Venice Blvd. Los Angeles, CA 90034

Pacific Women's Health Care 819 S. Vermont Ave. Los Angeles, CA 90005

Planned Parenthood 8520 So. Broadway Los Angeles, CA 90003

Planned Parenthood 1057 Kingston Ave. Los Angeles, CA 90033

Marina Women's Medical Group 4560 Admiralty Way, # 303 Marina Del Rey, CA 90292

Family Planning Assoc. Med. Grp. 10200 Sepulveda Blvd., # 200 Mission Hills, CA 91345

Family Planning Assoc. Med. Grp. 2030 Coffee Rd., # A1 Modesto, CA 95355

Family Planning Assoc. Med. Grp. 5050 San Bernardino St. Montclair, CA 91763

Planned Parenthood 225 San Antonio Rd. Mountain View, CA 94040

Family Planning Assoc. Med. Grp. 4501 Birch St., # 103 Newport Beach, CA 92660

Family Planning Specialists 200 Webster St., # 100 Oakland, CA 94607

Planned Parenthood 7200 Bancroft Ave., Ste. 210 Oakland, CA 94605

Family Planning Assoc. Med. Grp. 2445 W. Chapman Ave., # 200 Orange, CA 92868

Planned Parenthood 700 S. Tustin St. Orange, CA 92866

Her Medical Clinic 13309 Van Nuys Blvd. Pacoima, CA 91331

Planned Parenthood 1045 N. Lake Ave. Pasadena, CA 91104

Guerra Billie Yvonne Do 1456 Professional Dr Petaluma, CA 94954

Smith Forrest O MD 1393 Santa Rita Rd Pleasanton, CA 94566

Planned Parenthood 1550 N. Garey Ave. Pomona, CA 91767

Abortion Services 35400 Bob Hope Dr Suite 212 Rancho Mirage, CA 92270

Women's Health Specialists 1901 Victor Ave. Redding, CA 96002

Planned Parenthood 1230 Hopkins Ave. Redwood City, CA 94062

Health Care Center for Women 18905 Sherman Way, # 201 Reseda, CA 91335

Planned Parenthood 2970 Hilltop Mall Rd., # 307 Richmond, CA 94806

Family Planning Assoc. Med. Grp. 3660 Park Sierra Dr # 202 Riverside, CA 92501

Planned Parenthood 3772 Tibbetts St. Riverside, CA 92506

Planned Parenthood 1370 Medical Center Dr., Ste. E 2nd Fl. Rohnert Park, CA 94928

Family Planning Assoc. Med. Grp. 1280 San Gabriel Blvd. Rosemead, CA 91770

Planned Parenthood 729 Sunrise Ave., # 900 Roseville, CA 95661

Choice Medical Group 2322 Butano Dr., # 205 Sacramento, CA 95825

Planned Parenthood 201 29th St # B Sacramento, CA 95814

Pregnancy Consultation Center 5301 F St., # 10 Sacramento, CA 95819

Sacramento B Street Health Center 201 29th Street, Suite B Sacramento, CA 95816

Women's Health Specialists 1750 Wright St., Ste. 1 Sacramento, CA 95825

Choice Medical Group 945 Blanco Circle, # B Salinas, CA 93901

Family Planning Assoc. Med. Grp. 165 W. Hospitality Ln., # 1 San Bernardino, CA 92408

Planned Parenthood 1873 Commercenter W. San Bernardino, CA 92408

Dr. Robert Barmeyer 2929 Health Center Dr. San Diego, CA 92123

California Women's Medical Center 4134 Fairmont Ave. San Diego, CA 92105

Dr. Homer Chin-UCSD Women's Health Services 4168 Front St San Diego, CA 92103

Family Planning Assoc. Med. Grp., Dr. Robert Santella 7340 Miramar Road, Suite 205 San Diego, CA 92120

Planned Parenthood 2017 1st Ave, Ste 100 San Diego, CA 92101

San Diego Women's Medical Clinic aka California Women's Medical Clinic Dr. Michael Wong 4282 Genesee Ave., # 201 San Diego, CA 92117

217

Dr. Robert Santella 4531 College Ave San Diego, CA 92115

Choice Medical Group 2107 O'Farrell St. San Francisco, CA 94115

Mt. Zion Options Center 2356 Sutter St. San Francisco, CA 94115

Planned Parenthood 815 Eddy Street San Francisco, CA 94109

St. Luke's Women's Center Dr. Laura Norrell 1580 Valencia St. #508 San Francisco, CA 94110

Women's Options Center 1001 Potrero Ave., # 5 M San Francisco, CA 94110

Choice Medical Group 2365 Montpelier Dr. San Jose, CA 95116

Planned Parenthood 1691 The Alameda San Jose, CA 95126

Planned Parenthood 734 Pismo St. San Luis Obispo, CA 93401

North County Women's Medical Dr. George Kung 120 Craven Rd., # 209 San Marcos, CA 92078

Planned Parenthood 2211 Palm Ave. San Mateo, CA 94403

Planned Parenthood 2 H Street San Rafael, CA 94901

Abortion Services 120 W. 5th St., Ste. 100 Santa Ana, CA 92701

Alfa Primary Care Medical 405 Broadway Santa Ana, CA 92701

Family Planning Medical Clinic 1125 E. 17th St., #E108 Santa Ana, CA 92701

Planned Parenthood 518 Garden St. Santa Barbara, CA 93101

Planned Parenthood 1119 Pacific Ave., # 200 Santa Cruz, CA 95060

Planned Parenthood 415 E. Chapel St. Santa Maria, CA 93454

Women's Health Specialists 4415 Sonoma Hwy., # D Santa Rosa, CA 95409

Planned Parenthood of Monterey 625 Hilby Ave. Seaside, CA 93955

Her Smart Choice/Clinica Los Remedios Dr. Vikram Kothandaraman 4835 Van Nuys Blvd. Ste 203 Sherman Oaks, CA 91403

Simi Women's Center 2840 E. Los Angeles Ave. Simi Valley, CA 93065

North Planned Parenthood 415 W Benjamin Holt Dr., # D2 Stockton, CA 95207

Stockton Pregnancy Control 3209 N. California St. Stockton, CA 95204

Planned Parenthood 166 North Moorpark Rd. Ste. 104 Thousand Oaks, CA 91360

Family Planning Assoc. Med. Grp. 3655 Lomita Blvd., #400 Torrance, CA 90505

Women's Care Center 18051 Crenshaw Blvd., # C Torrance, CA 90504

Planned Parenthood 990 Broadway St. Vallejo, CA 94590

Planned Parenthood 7100 Van Nuys Blvd., # 108 Van Nuys, CA 91505

Van Nuys Women's Care 7232 Van Nuys Blvd., # 101 Van Nuys, CA 91405

Planned Parenthood 5400 Ralston St. Ventura, CA 93003

Planned Parenthood 1357 Oakland Blvd. Walnut Creek, CA 94596

Confidential Care 22110 Roscoe Blvd., # 203 West Hills, CA 91304

Westwind Women's Services/Abortions by Choice 22110 Roscoe Blvd., # 104 West Hills, CA 91304

Family Planning Assoc. Med. Grp. 12304 Santa Monica, # 112 West Los Angeles, CA 90025

Pro-Choice Med. Ctr. Dr. Josepha Seletz 10150 National Blvd. West Los Angeles, CA 90034

Planned Parenthood 7655 Greenleaf Ave. Whittier, CA 90602

COLORADO – 16 Locations

Mayfair Women's Center 14446 E. Evans Ave. Aurora, CO 80014

Boulder Abortion Clinic Dr. Warren Hern 1130 Alpine Ave. Boulder, CO 80304

Boulder Valley Women's Health Ctr. 2855 Valmont Rd. Boulder, CO 80301

Planned Parenthood of the Rocky Mtns. 1330 W. Colorado Ave. Colorado Springs, CO 80904

Abortion Access Dr. Bernstein 1295 Colorado Blvd. Denver, CO 80206

Abortion Counseling Service 1340 Leyden St. Denver, CO 80220

Fertility & Family Planning 4500 E. 9th Ave., # 700 Denver, CO 80220

Ob/Gyn, Dr. O'Loughlin & Dr. Rosewater 850 E. Harvard Ave., Suite 565 Denver, CO 80210

Mile High Ob Gyn 455 S Hudson St Floor 2 Denver, CO 80246

Planned Parenthood 7155 E 38th Ave Denver, CO 80207

Women's Care Dr. Arthur Waldbaum 1201 E. 17th Ave, Suite 200 Denver, CO 80218

Planned Parenthood 46 Suttle St. Durango, CO 81303

Healthy Futures For Women Dr. Stephen Hindes 300 East Hampden Ave., Ste. 201 Englewood, CO 80113

Mile High Ob Gyn 8200 East Belleview, Suite 320 Englewood, CO 80111

Mountain Vista Women's Care 701 E. Hampden Ave. Ste. 110 Englewood, CO 80113

Abortion Counseling Assoc. 181 W. Meadow Dr., # 200 Vail, CO 81657

CONNECTICUT – 9 Locations

Summit Women's Center 3787 Main St. Bridgeport, CT 06606

Medical Options 27 Hospital Ave. Suite 202 Danbury, CT 06810

Womancare & Teencare 27 Hospital Ave. Danbury, CT 06810

Hartford GYN Center 1 Main St., # N1 Hartford, CT 06106

Summit Women's Center 360 Market St. Hartford, CT 06120

Planned Parenthood 345 Whitney Ave New Haven, CT 06511

Planned Parenthood 12 Case St., # 213 Nowrich, CT 06360

Planned Parenthood 1039 E. Main St. Stamford, CT 06902

Planned Parenthood 1030 New Britain Ave. West Hartford, CT 06110

DELAWARE – 4 Locations

Atlantic Women's Medical 1643 N. DuPont Hwy. Dover, DE 19901

Planned Parenthood 805 S. Governors Ave. Dover, DE 19904

Atlantic Women's Medical 2809 Baynard Blvd. Wilmington, DE 19802

Planned Parenthood 625 N. Shipley St. Wilmington, DE 19801

District of Columbia – 4 Locations

Planned Parenthood 1108 16th St. NW Washington, DC 20036

Potomac Family Planning Center 3230 Pennsylvania Ave. SE, #200 Washington, DC 20020

Southeast Women's Health Center 3794 M.L. King Jr. Ave SE, # 100 Washington, DC 20032

Washington Surgi-Center 2112 F. Street NW, Suite 400 Washington, DC 20037

FLORIDA – 69 Locations

All Women's Health Center 431 Maitland Ave Altamonte Springs, FL 32701

Bread and Roses 1560 S Highland Ave Clearwater, FL 33756

Women's OB/GYN of Countryside 28960 US Highway 19 N., Suite 110 Clearwater, FL 33761

Gynecologic Surgeons 2929 N University Dr. # 202 Coral Springs, FL 33065

Woman's Health/Birth Control Ctr Inc 1225 8th St. Daytona Beach, FL 32117

Women's Awareness 5700 Griffin Rd # 130 Davie, FL 33314

All Women's Center 2100 E. Commercial Blvd Fort Lauderdale, FL 33308

Dr. Benjamin 7777 N. University Dr. #102 Fort Lauderdale, FL 33321

Ft. Lauderdale Women's Center 2001 W. Oakland Park Blvd. Fort Lauderdale, FL 33311

Today's Woman Medical Center 6971 W Sunrise Blvd. # 206 Fort Lauderdale, FL 33313

Women's Center 962 E Cypress Creek Rd. Fort Lauderdale, FL 33334

Ft. Myers Women's Health Center 3900 Broadway Blvd., Bldg. C Fort Myers, FL 33901

Planned Parenthood 8595 College Parkway, Suite 250 Ft. Myers, FL 33919

Southwest Florida Women's Clinic Dr. Ali A. Azima 710 Pondella Rd. # 12 Fort Myers, FL 33903

A Woman's World Medical Center 503 S. 12th St. Fort Pierce, FL 34950

All Women's Health Center Inc 1135 NW 23rd Ave., Suite N Gainesville, FL 32609

Bread and Roses Women's Health 1233 NW 10th Ave Gainesville, FL 32601

A GYN Diagnostic Center 267 E. 49th St. Hialeah, FL 33013

Alba Medical Clinic 4210 Palm Ave. Hialeah, FL 33012

A Women's Care II 952 E. 25th St. Hialeah, FL 33013

A Woman's Choice 6406 NW 186th St. Hialeah, FL 33015

A Woman's Option Inc. 1933 W. 60th St. Hialeah, FL 33012

Woman's A Center of Hollywood 3829 Hollywood Blvd # D Hollywood, FL 33021

A Jacksonville Women's Health 4131 University Blvd. S., Build. # 2 Jacksonville, FL 32216

All Florida Women's Center 3599 University Blvd. S # 1200 Jacksonville, FL 32216

All Women's Clinic 4331 University Blvd. S Jacksonville, FL 32216

Savannah Medical Clinic 120 E 34th St Savannah Jacksonville, FL 32201

Lakeland Women's Health Center 4444 S Florida Ave. Lakeland, FL 33813

Advanced Gyn Clinic 6464 N Miami Ave Miami, FL 33150

A Eve Center Dr. Gerald Applegate 3900 NW 79th Ave., # 575 Miami, FL 33166

A Eve of Kendall 8603 South Dixie Highway Kendall 1 Plaza, Suite102 Miami, FL 33143

A Woman's Care 68 NE 167th St., # A Miami, FL 33162

Blue Coral Women's Care Inc 7360 Coral Way # 16 Miami, FL 33155

Department of Obstetrics and Gynecology 1321 NW 14 Street, #201 Miami, FL 33136

Millennium Women Center Inc 9370 SW 72nd St # A104 Miami, FL 33173

New World Medical Choice 2036 SW 1st St. Rear Miami, FL 33135

Today's Women's Medical Center 3250 S Dixie HWY Miami, FL 33133

Top-GYN Ladies Center 44 W Flager St. Miami, FL 33134

Women's Health Care Inc 1250 SW 1st St. Miami, FL 33135

Gynecologists Diagnostic Center 6161 Miramar PKWY Miramar, FL 33023

Planned Parenthood 1425 Creech Road Naples, FL 34103

Today's Woman Medical Center 909 NE 163rd St. # 402 North Miami Beach, FL 33162

Women & Teens Community Health 16876 NE 19th Ave. North Miami Beach, FL 33162

Ocala Women's Center 108 NW Pine Ave. Ocala, FL 34475

WomanCare /Abortion Center 4574 E. Michigan St. Orlando, FL 32812

EPOC Clinic 609 Virginia Dr. Orlando, FL 32803

Orlando Women's Center 1103 Lucerne Terrace Orlando, FL 32806

Planned Parenthood of Greater Orlando 726 S. Tampa Ave. Orlando, FL 32805

Pensacola Medical Services 6115 Village Oaks Dr. Pensacola, FL 32504

Aastra 10 SW 44th Ave Plantation, FL 33317

All Women's OB/GYN Group 817 S University Dr. # 101 Plantation, FL 33324

Today's Woman Medical Centers 6971 W Sunrise Blvd Ste 206 Plantation, FL 33313

Venice Woman's Health Center 21178 Olean Blvd. # C Port Charlotte, FL 33952

All Women's Clinic 2700 S. Tamiami Trail, # 5 Sarasota, FL 34239

Planned Parenthood 736 Central Ave. Sarasota, FL 34236

A Choice for Women 6660 S. West 117th Ave. South Miami, FL 33143

All Women's Center 4131 Central Ave St. Petersburg, FL 33713

Planned Parenthood 10051 5th Street North, #109 St. Petersburg, FL 33702

Women's Health Center 3401 66th St. N St. Petersburg, FL 33710

N. FL Women's Hlth & Counseling 1345 Cross Creek Way Tallahas., FL 32301

BSSI, Dr. Michael Benjamin 7707 N. University Dr., # 206 Tamarac, FL 33321

All Women's Clinic 14401 Bruce B Downs Blvd. Tampa, FL 33613

All Women's Health Center 3330 W Kennedy Blvd. Tampa, FL 33609

Tampa Women's Health Center 2010 E Fletcher Ave. Tampa, FL 33612

Women's Center of Hyde Park 502 S Magnolia Ave. Tampa, FL 33606

Presidential Women's Center 100 N Point Parkway West Palm Beach, FL 33407

Planned Parenthood 908 Spring Lake Square Winter Haven, FL 33881

GEORGIA – 14 Locations

Atlanta SurgiCenter – Piedmont Pointe Complex 1874 Piedmont Road, Suite #580 E Atlanta, GA 30324

Atlanta Women's Medical Center 235 W. Wieuca Rd. NE Atlanta, GA 30342

Dunwoody Women's Medical Group 3114 Mercer University St. # 100 Atlanta, GA 30341

Feminist Women's Health Center 1924 Cliff Valley Way NE Atlanta, GA 30329

Northside Women's Clinic 3543 Chamblee-Dunwoody Rd. Atlanta, GA 30341

Summit Medical Assoc. 1874 Piedmont Rd. NE, # 500 E Atlanta, GA 30324

A Preferred Women's Health Center 2903 Professional PKWY Augusta, GA 30907

Planned Parenthood 1289 Broad St. Augusta, GA 30901

Old National Gynecology 6210 Old National Hwy College Park, GA 30349

National Women's Health 3850 Rosemont Dr. Columbus, GA 31904

Dekalb Gynecology Assoc. 4229 Snapfinger Woods Dr. Decatur, GA 30035

AB Services 1640 Powers Ferry Rd. SE, Building 23 Marietta, GA 30067

North Georgia Family Planning 11205 Alpharetta Hwy # 2 Roswell, GA 30076

Abortion Clinic of Savannah 120 E. 34th St. Savannah, GA 31401

HAWAII – 3 Locations

Planned Parenthood of Hawaii 1350 S King St. # 310 Honolulu, HI 96814

Planned Parenthood – Kahului Clinic 140 Hoohana Street, Suite 303 Kahului, HI 96732

Planned Parenthood of Hawaii 75-184 Hualalai Rd. # 205 Kailua Kona, HI 96740

IDAHO – 2 Locations

Planned Parenthood 3668 N. Harbor Lane Boise, ID 83703

Dr. Glenn Weyhrich 222 N 2nd St. Boise, ID 83702

ILLINOIS – 22 Locations

Planned Parenthood Aurora Health Center 3051 East New York Street Aurora, IL 60504

Women's Health Practice 2125 N Neil St. Champaign, IL 61820

All Women's Health Chicago 2000 W. Armitage Avenue Chicago, IL 60647

American Women's Center 2744 N Western Ave. Chicago, IL 60647

Fam. Planning Assoc. Med. Group 659 W Washington Blvd. Chicago, IL 60661

Fam. Planning Assoc. Med. Group 5086 N Elston Ave. Chicago, IL 60630

Medical Group 7845 S Cottage Grove Ave. #104 Chicago, IL 60619

Michigan Avenue Center for Health 2415 S. Michigan Ave Chicago, IL 60616

Planned Parenthood 1200 N La Salle Dr. Chicago, IL 60610

Ryan Center at University of Chicago 5758 S. Maryland Ave. Chicago, IL 60637

The UIC Center for Reproductive Health *Abortion location undisclosed* Chicago, IL

American Women's Center 110 S River Rd Suite 7 Des Plaines, IL 60016

Dimensions Medical Center Ltd. 1455 E Golf Rd. # 108 Des Plaines, IL 60016

Forest View Medical Center 2750 South River Road Des Plaines, IL 60018

Access Health Center 1700 75th St. Downers Grove, IL 60516

Aanchor Health Center Ltd. Dr. Goyal 1186 Roosevelt Rd. Glen Ellyn, IL 60137

The Hope Clinic for Women Dr. Yogendra Shah 1602 21st St. Granite City, IL 62040

ACU Health Center Ltd. 736 N. York Rd. Hinsdale, IL 60521

Women's Aid Clinic 4751 W Touhy Ave. #101 Lincolnwood, IL 60646

National Health Care 7405 N University St. Peoria, IL 61614

Northern IL Women's Center 1400 Broadway # 201 Rockford, IL 61104

Advantage Health Care Ltd. 203 E Irving Park Rd. Wood Dale, IL 60191

INDIANA – 10 Locations

Planned Parenthood 421 S College Ave. Bloomington, IN 47403

Ft. Wayne Women's Health Organization 2210 Inwood Drive Ft. Wayne, IN 46815

Indiana Women's Center 916 W. Coliseum Blvd. #8 Fort Wayne, IN 46808

Friendship Family Planning 3700 Broadway Gary, IN 46408

Affiliated Women's Services 2215 Distributors Dr. Indianapolis, IN 46242

Clinic for Women 3607 W 16th St. # 2 B Indianapolis, IN 46218

Indianapolis Women's Center 1201 N Arlington Ave. # D Indianapolis, IN 46219

Planned Parenthood 8590 Georgetown Road Indianapolis, IN 46268

Planned Parenthood of Greater Indiana 8645 Connecticut St. Merrillville, IN 46410

Women's Pavilion 2010 Ironwood Circle South Bend, IN 46635

IOWA - 5 Locations

Planned Parenthood 2751 Tech Dr. Bettendorf, IA 52722

Planned Parenthood 1000 East Army Post Road Des Moines, IA 50315

Emma Goldman Clinic 227 N. Dubuque St. Iowa City, IA 52245

Planned Parenthood 850 Orchard St. Iowa City, IA 52246

Planned Parenthood 4409 Stone Ave. Sioux City, IA 51106

KANSAS - 3 Locations

Abortion Access For Women Dr. Ronald Yoemans 720 Central Ave. Kansas City, KS 66101

Center for Women's Health Dr. Herbert Hodes, Dr. Tracy Nauser (father/daughter abortionist team) 4840 College Blvd. Overland Park, KS 66211

Planned Parenthood Comprehensive Health 4401 W. 109th St. Overland Park, KS 66211

KENTUCKY - 2 Locations

EMW Women's Clinic 161 Burt Rd. Lexington, KY 40503

EMW Women's Surgical Center 138 W Market St. Louisville, KY 40202

LOUISIANA - 7 Locations

Delta Clinic 756 Colonial Dr # B Baton Rouge, LA 70806

Abortion Assistance 1505 Doctors Dr. Bossier City, LA 71111

Causeway Medical Suite 3040 Ridgelake Drive Metairie, LA 70002

Causeway Medical Clinic 2701 General Pershing New Orleans, LA 70015

East Women's Clinic 3500 St Charles Ave New Orleans, LA 70115

Gentilly Medical Clinic 3030 Gentilly Blvd. New Orleans, LA 70122

Hope Medical Group for Women 210 Kings HWY Shreveport, LA 71104

225

MAINE – 4 Locations

Family Planning Assn. Of Maine 43 Gabriel Dr. Augusta, ME 04332

Mabel Wadsworth Women's Health Center 700 Mount Hope Avenue Bangor, ME 04401

Planned Parenthood 970 Forest Ave. Portland, ME 04104

Family Planning Associates 92 Darling Ave. South Portland, ME 04106

MARYLAND – 23 Locations

Planned Parenthood 929 West St. Annapolis, MD 21401

American Health Care Services 3506 N. Calvert St., Ste. 110 Baltimore, MD 21218

Gynemed Surgi-Center 17 Fontana Lane # 201 Baltimore, MD 21237

Hillcrest Clinic of Baltimore 5602 Baltimore National Pike # 600 Baltimore, MD 21228

Planned Parenthood 330 N Howard St. Baltimore, MD 21201

Whole Women's Health Baltimore 7648 Belair Rd. Baltimore, MD 21236

Wisconsin Ave Women's Center 8311 Wisconsin Ave. # C14 Bethesda, MD 20814

Annapolis Medical Center Dr. Aalai 6532 Annapolis Rd. Ste. 7 Bladensburg, MD 20710

American Women's Services 4700 Berwin House Rd., Ste. 203 College Park, MD 20740

Metropolitan Fam. Planning Institute 5915 Greenbelt Rd. College Park, MD 20740

American Women's Services 801 Toll House Ave., Unit H6 Fredrick, MD 21701

Integrated OB/GYN Services 7610 Pennsylvania Ave #305 Forestville, MD 20747

Women's Health Care Center 9061 Shady Grove Ct Gaithersburg, MD 20877

Metropolitan Fam. Planning Institute 9063 Shady Grove Court Gaithersburg, MD 20877

Germantown Reprod. Hlth Srvcs 13233 Executive Park Terrace Germantown, MD 20874

Hagerstown Reproductive Health Services 160 W Washington St Hagerstown, MD 21740

MD Women's Abortion Clinic 6005 Landover Rd. # 6 Hyattsville, MD 20785

Prince George's Repro. Hlth. Srvcs. 7411 Riggs Rd. # 300 Hyattsville, MD 20783

Femi-Care Surgery Center 66 Painters Mill Rd. Owings Mills, MD 21117

Potomac Family Planning Center 966 Hungerford Dr. # 24 Rockville, MD 20850

Gyncare Center 877 Baltimore Annapolis # 300 Severna Park, MD 21146

Planned Parenthood of Metropolitian DC 1400 Spring St. Silver Spring, MD 20910

Metropolitan Fam. Planning Institute 5625 Allentown Rd. # 203 Suitland, MD 20746

MASSACHUSETTS - 12 Locations

Four Women 152 Emory St. Attleboro, MA 02703

Planned Parenthood League of MA 1055 Commonwealth Ave. Boston, MA 02215

Office of Boris I. Orkin 1180 Beacon Street, Suite 5b Brookline, MA 02446

Office of Shaio Yu-Lee 1180 Beacon St. Suite 7A Brookline, MA 02446

Women's' Health Services 111 Harvard St. Brookline MA 02446

Atlanticare OB/GYN 9 Boston St. FL 3 Lynn, MA 01904

North Shore Women's Center 480 Lynnfield St. FL 2 Lynn, MA 01904

Merrimack Valley Women's Health 288 Groveland St. Haverhill, MA 01830

Office of Nicholas Pantelakis 6 Essex Center Dr.,# 201 Peabody, MA 01960

Planned Parenthood of Western MA 3550 Main Street Springfield, MA 01107

Suburban Women's Health 241 Boston Post Rd Wayland, MA 02144

Planned Parenthood 470 Pleasant Street Worcester, MA 01609

MICHIGAN - 33 Locations

Planned Parenthood 3100 Professional Dr. Ann Arbor, MI 48104

Health Care Clinic Inc. 3012 Packard St. Ann Arbor, MI 48108

Women's Advisory Center 43700 Woodward Ave/ # 104 Bloomfield TWP, MI 48302

Northland Family Planning Center 41700 Hayes Rd. # B Clinton TWP, MI 48038

American Family Planning Inc 4132 Schaefer Rd. Dearborn, MI 48126

Detroit/Grosse Pointe Sharpe Family Planning 16738 E. Warren Detroit, MI 48224

East GYN Women's Center 15650 E 8 Mile Rd. Detroit, MI 48205

Scottsdale Women's Center 19305 W 7 Mile Rd. Detroit, MI 48219

Summit Medical Center 15801 W McNichols Rd. Detroit, MI 48235

Feminine Health Care Clinic 2032 S Saginaw St. Flint, MI 48503

Women's Health Center G 3422 Flushing Rd. Flint, MI 48504

Heritage Clinic for Women 320 Fulton NE Grand Rapids, MI 49503

Women's Medical Center 3212 Eastern Ave. SE Grand Rapids, MI 49508

Planned Parenthood 4201 W Michigan Ave. Kalamazoo, MI 49006

WomansChoice 6500 Centurion Dr # 290 Lansing, MI 48912

Womancare of Lansing 1601 E Grand River Ave Ste D Lansing, MI 48906

Women's Medical Services 863 E Apple Ave. Muskegon, MI 49442

Michiana Abortion Clinic 703 E Main St. Niles, MI 49120

WomansChoice 3141 Cabaret Trail S., # 400 Saginaw, MI 48603

Women's Health Center 3141 Cabaret Trail S # 100 Saginaw, MI 48603

Northland Fam. Plan. Ctr. West 24450 Evergreen Road STE 220 Southfield, MI 48075

Physician's Abortion Services 29425 Northwestern HWY # 125 Southfield, MI 48034

Womancare of Southfield 28505 Southfield Rd. Southfield, MI 48076

Womancare of Downriver 14523 Northline Rd. Southgate, MI 48195

Birth Control Center 2783 E 14 Mile Rd. Sterling Heights, MI 48310

Northland Family Planning 37300 Dequindre, Suite 102 Sterling Heights, MI 48310

Womancare Inc. 11474 15 Mile Rd. Sterling Heights, MI 48312

Women's Center 28477 Hoover Road Warren, MI 48093

Womens Clinic Group 2665 Elizabeth Lake Rd., # 104 Waterford, MI 48328

Women's Center 6765 Orchard Lake Rd. West Bloomfield, MI 48322

Northland Fam. Plan. Ctr. West 35000 Ford Rd. Westland, MI 48185

MINNESOTA – 7 Locations

Women's Health Center 32 E. 1st # 300 Duluth, MN 55802

Dr. Mildred Hanson-Medical Aids 710 E 24th St. # 403 Minneapolis, MN 55404

Meadowbrook Women's Clinic 825 S 8th St. # 1018 Minneapolis, MN 55404

228

Midwest Health Center For Women 33 S 5th St. FL 4 Minneapolis, MN 55402

Robbinsdale Clinic 3819 W Broadway Ave. Robbinsdale, MN 55422

GYN Special Services 640 Jackson Street St. Paul, MN 55101

Highland Park Planned Parenthood 1965 Ford Pkwy. St. Paul, MN 55116

MISSISSIPPI – 1 Location

Jackson Women's Health Org. 2903 N. State St. Jackson, MS 39216

MISSOURI – 3 Locations

Women's Care GYN Inc 3394 McElvey Rd. # 111 Bridgeton, MO 63044

Planned Parenthood 711 N Providence Rd. Columbia, MO 65203

Central West End Planned Parenthood 4251 Forest PKWY St. Louis, MO 63108

MONTANA – 5 Locations

Planned Parenthood Heights 100 West Wicks Lane Billings, MT 59105

Planned Parenthood 1500 Cannon St. Helena, MT 59601

All Families Healthcare 1060 N Meridian Rd Kalispell, MT 59901

Mountain Country Women's Clinic Dr. Susan Wicklund 207 South Main Street Livingston, MT 59047

Blue Mountain Clinic 610 N California St. Missoula, MT 59802

NEBRASKA – 2 Locations

Abortion Contraception Clinic of NE Dr. LeRoy Carhart 1002 W Mission Ave. Bellevue, NE 68005

Planned Parenthood Dr. C.J. LaBenz 3705 South St. Lincoln, NE 68506

NEVADA – 7 Locations

Green Valley Abortion Services 1701 N Green Valley Pkwy #3-B Henderson, NV 89074

AAA Abortions 3700 E Charleston Blvd Las Vegas, NV 89104

A-All Women Care 3599 S. Eastern Avenue Las Vegas, NV 89169

A to Z Women's Center Dr. Ramos/ Dr. Levy 1670 E Flamingo Rd. # C Las Vegas, NV 89119

Birth Control Care Ctr Dr. Meeger 872 E Sahara Ave. Las Vegas, NV 89104

Abortion Services 2031 McDaniel St., # 240 North Las Vegas, NV 89030

West End Women's Medical Group Dr. Damon Suites 5915 Tyrone Rd. Reno, NV 89502

NEW HAMPSHIRE - 5 Locations

Concord Feminist Health Center 38 S Main St. Concord, NH 03301

Feminist Health Ctr of Portsmouth 559 Portsmouth Ave. Greenland, NH 03840

Manchester Obstetrical Associates 150 Tarrytown Road Manchester, NH 03103

Planned Parenthood 24 Pennacook Street Manchester, NH 03104

Planned Parenthood 89 S. Main St. West Lebanon, NH 03784

NEW JERSEY - 28

Atlantic Womens Health 707 White Horse Pike # A4 Absecon, NJ 08201

Cherry Hill Women's Center 502 Kings Hwy. N. Cherry Hill, NJ 08034

South Jersey Women's Center 1014 Haddonfield Rd. Cherry Hill, NJ 08002

E. Brunswick Women's Center 5 Cornwall Ct., # B4 East Brunswick, NJ 08816

Women's Services 112 S. Munn Ave. East Orange, NJ 07018

Associates in Ob. & Gyn. 700 N. Broad Street Elizabeth, NJ 07208

Abortion Center of Englewood 200 Grand Ave # 101 Englewood, NJ 07631

Comprehensive Women's Care 401 S. Van Brunt St. #405 Englewood, NJ 07631

Metropolitan Medical Assoc. 40 Engle St. Englewood, NJ 07631

Abortion Service of Fort Lee 2231 Lemoine Ave. Fort Lee, NJ 07024

Women's Choice 10 Zabriskie St. Hackensack, NJ 07601

Options 102 Candlewood Commons Howell, NJ 07731

Dr. Kenneth Chang 3144 John F. Kennedy Blvd. Jersey City, NJ 07305

Pilgrim Medical Center Inc. 393 Bloomfield Ave. Montclair, NJ 07042

American Women's Services 3 Winslow Pl., Fl. 2 Paramus, NJ 07652

American Women's Services 157 S Main St. Phillipsburg, NJ 08865

Options Gynesurgical Assoc. 1024 Park Ave #4 Plainfield, NJ 07060

Princeton Women's Center 29 Emmons Dr., # E-20 Princeton, NJ 08540

Chang Kenneth S MD 605 Broad Ave, Ste 201 Ridgefield, NJ 07657

Planned Parenthood 69 Newman Springs Rd. Shrewsbury, NJ 07702

Robert Levitt, MD 516 Easton Ave. Somerset, NJ 08873

American Women's Services 651 Route 37 West Tom's River, NJ 08755

Planned Parenthood 437 E State St. Trenton, NJ 08608

Women's Medical Center 2406 Bergenline Union, NJ 07087

Union Ob/Gyn 1323 Stuyvesant Ave. Union, NJ 07083

American Women's Services 1 Alpha Ave., Ste. 27 Voorhees, NJ 08043

South Orange Women's Care LLC 737 Northfield Ave West Orange, NJ 07052

American Women's Services 228 Main St. Woodbridge, NJ 07095

NEW MEXICO - 5 Locations

Southwestern Women's Options (AKA Abortion Acceptance of New Mexico) Dr. Curtis Boyd 522 Lomas Blvd NE Albuquerque, NM 87102

Dr. Bruce Ferguson 1101 Medical Arts Ave. NE, # B Albuquerque, NM 87102

Planned Parenthood 701 San Mateo Blvd. NE Albuquerque, NM 87108

Dr. Lucia Cies 435 Saint Michaels Dr., # B-201 Santa Fe, NM 87505

Hilltop Women's Reproductive Clinic Dr. Theard 5690 Santa Teresita Dr. Santa Teresa, NM 88008

NEW YORK - 82 Locations

Planned Parenthood 259 Lark St. Albany, NY 12210

Michael Afshari 216-04 Union Turnpike Bayside, NY 11364

Planned Parenthood 395 Main St. Beacon, NY 12508

Bronx Women's Health 1100 Pelham Pkwy. S. Bronx, NY 10461

Bronx Women's Medical Services Dr. Robert Hosty 2901 3rd Ave. FL 2 Bronx, NY 10455

Dr. Emily's Women's Health Center 560 Southern Blvd Bronx, NY 10455

Gyns Management Services aka Gynecological Surgical Services 2070 Eastchester Rd. Bronx, NY 10461

Lincoln Medical Center 234 East 149 St. Bronx, NY 10451

Metropolitan Health Center 2330 Grand Concourse Bronx, NY 10461

Planned Parenthood 349 E. 149th St. Bronx, NY 10451

A Brooklyn Woman's Medical 44 Court St. # 322 Brooklyn, NY 11201

Ambulatory Surgery Center 313 43rd St. Brooklyn, NY 11232

Brooklyn Women's Services Dr. Salomon Epstein 6721 Avenue U Brooklyn, NY 11234

Early Options/ Women and Family Health Dr. Joan Fleischman, Dr. Judy Washington 188 Montague St. Ste 404 Brooklyn, NY 11201

Planned Parenthood 44 Court St. 6th Floor Brooklyn, NY 11201

The Women's Choice Robert E. Rainer 81 Willoughby St. Ste. 601 Brooklyn, NY 11201

Wyckoff Heights Medical Center 110 Wycoff Ave. Room 118 Brooklyn, NY 11237

Planned Parenthood 2505 Carmel Ave Brewster, NY 10509

Buffalo GYN Women's Services 2500 Main St. Buffalo, NY 14214

Dr. Shalom Press 2550 Sweet Home Rd. Buffalo, NY 14226

Planned Parenthood 23 Main St. Cobleskill, NY 12043

Begum Firoza 123 Grant Ave East Rockaway, NY 11518

Abortion Information & Services 6602 Franklin Park Dr. East Syracuse, NY 13057

Women's Health Horizons 824 Franklin Park Dr. East Syracuse, NY 13057

lmhurst Women's Medical Care 40-24 76th St. Elmhurst, NY 11373

Planned Parenthood Elmira Center 755 East Church Street Elmira, NY 14901

Abortion Women's Medical 3713 85th St. FL 1 Flushing, NY 11372

Forest Hill Woman's Services 10816 63rd Rd. Flushing, NY 11375

Liberty Women's Health Care 3701 Main St. # 500 Flushing, NY 11354

Dr. Linda Kim 3730 73rd St Flushing, NY 11372

New York OB/GYN Assoc 9229 Queens Blvd. # CA Flushing, NY 11374

Professional Women's Services Inc. 8926 Roosevelt Ave. Flushing, NY 11217

All Women's Medical Pavilion 6930 Austin St. Forest Hills, NY 11375

Glen Cove Planned Parenthood 110 School Street Glen Cove, NY 11542

Planned Parenthood 135 Warren St. Glen Falls, NY 12801

Planned Parenthood 7 Coates Drive, Suite 4 Goshen, NY 10924

Women's Choice 200 Motor Pkwy Hauppauge, NY 11788

Planned Parenthood of Nassau 540 Fulton Ave. Hempstead, NY 11550

Planned Parenthood 190 Fairview Ave. Hudson, NY 12534

Medical Offices of P.P. 314 W State St. Ithaca, NY 14850

Roosevelt Women's Med Care 78-13 Roosevelt Ave. Jackson Heights, NY 11372

Women's Services Dr. Salomon Epstein 37-54 75th St Jackson Heights, NY 11372

Comprehensive Women's Health Dr. Mahendranauth Sohan 10612 Liberty Ave. Jamaica, NY 11417

Planned Parenthood 169 Washington Avenue Kingston, NY 12401

Choices Women's Medical Center Dr. Evans Crevecoeur, Dr. George McMillan 2928 41st Ave. Long Island, NY 11101

All Womens Care 444 Community Dr. Manhasset, NY 11030

South Orange GYN 600 Route 208 Monroe, NY 10950

Planned Parenthood 14 Prince Street Monticello, NY 12701

Planned Parenthood 247 North Ave. New Rochelle, NY 10801

Planned Parenthood 532 Blooming Grove Tpke. New Windsor, NY 12553

Dr. Beitner 211 Central Park W. New York, NY 10024

Dr. Wong's Women's Health 110 Lafayette St. #502 New York, NY 10013

Early Options/ Women and Family Health Dr. Joan Fleischman, Dr. Judy Washington 124 E. 40th St. Ste 702 New York, NY 10019

Eastside Gynecology Assoc 225 E. 64th St. # C New York, NY 10001

Empire Women's Care 38 W. 32nd St. # 601 New York, NY 10001

Dr. Ahmed Fahmy 161 Madison Ave #2W New York, NY 10016

Manhattan Woman's Medical 461 Park Avenue S. 11th floor New York, NY 10022

Parkmed Eastern Women's Center 800 Second Avenue – 7th Floor New York, NY 10017

Phillips Family Practice 16 East 16th St. – 1st floor New York, NY 10003

Planned Parenthood 26 Bleecker St. New York, NY 10012

Westside Women's Medical Center Dr. Gluck 1841 Broadway # 1011 New York, NY 10023

Womens Comprehensive Health/ Dr. Kurt Christopher 48 E 43rd St New York, NY 10017

Planned Parenthood – Wheatfield 6951 Williams Road Niagara Falls, NY 14304

Northern Adirondack P.P. 66 Brinkerhoff St. Plattsburgh, NY 12901

Planned Parenthood 17 Noxon St. Poughkeepsie, NY 12601

Center for Menstrual Disorders & Reproductive Choice Dr. Wortman 2020 S. Clinton Ave. Rochester, NY 14618

Freedom of Choice 125 Lattimore Rd Suite 280 Rochester, NY 14620

Planned Parenthood 114 University Ave. Rochester, NY 14605

South Avenue Women's Services 990 South Av. Ste. 104A Rochester, NY 14620

Planned Parenthood 1040 State St. Schenectady, NY 12307

Planned Parenthood 70 Maple Ave. Smithtown, NY 11787

Stony Brook Women's Health Svc Dr. David Shobin 498 Route 111 Smithtown, NY 11787

Planned Parenthood 25 Perlman Drive at Pascack Plaza Spring Valley, NY 10977

Planned Parenthood 1120 E Genesee St. Syracuse, NY 13210

Planned Parenthood 200 Broadway, 3rd Flr. Troy, NY 12180

Planned Parenthood 1424 Genesee St. Utica, NY 13502

Southern Tier Women's Services Dr. Cousins 149 Vestal PKWY W Vestal, NY 13851

All Women's Health & Medical Srvcs. 222 Mamaroneck Ave. White Plains, NY 10605

Planned Parenthood 175 Tarrytown Rd. White Plains, NY 10601

Planned Parenthood 20 South Broadway Yonkers, NY 10701

Women's Health Resource 1990 Central Park Ave. Yonkers, NY 10710

NORTH CAROLINA – 17 Locations

Femcare 62 Orange St. Asheville, NC 28801

Eastowne OB-GYN & Infertility 180 Providence Rd. # 3 Chapel Hill, NC 27514

Planned Parenthood 1765 Dobbins Dr. Chapel Hill, NC 27514

Carolina Center For Women 421 N Wendover Rd. Charlotte, NC 28211

Family Reproductive Health 700 E. Hebron St. Charlotte, NC 28273

Preferred Women's Health Center 3220 Latrobe Dr. Charlotte, NC 28211

Carolina Women's Medical Clinic 1919 Gillespie St. Fayetteville, NC 29306

Planned Parenthood 4551 Yadkin Rd Fayetteville, NC 28303

A Woman's Choice 201 Pomona Dr. # E Greensboro, NC 27407

Piedmont Carolina Medical Clinic 2425 Randleman Rd. Greensboro, NC 27406

Abortion Services 712 N Elm St High Point, NC 27262

Crist Clinic for Women 250 Memorial Drive Jacksonvillle, NC 28546

A Preferred Health Center 1604 Jones Franklin Rd. Raleigh, NC 27606

A Woman's Choice 3305 Drake Circle Raleigh, NC 27607

Raleigh Women's Health Organization 3613 Haworth Dr. Raleigh, NC 27609

Planned Parenthood 1925 Tradd Ct. Wilmington, NC 28401

Planned Parenthood 3000 Maplewood Ave. Winston Salem, NC 27103

NORTH DAKOTA – 1 Location

Red River Women's Clinic 512 1st Ave. North North Fargo, ND 58102

OHIO – 16 Locations

Akron Women's Medical Group 839 E Market St. Akron, OH 44305

Planned Parenthood 2314 Auburn Ave. Cincinnatti, OH 45219

Women's Medical Center Dr. Martin Haskell 3219 Jefferson Ave. Cincinnati, OH 45220

Cleveland Surgi-Center 4269 Pearl Rd. Ste. 406 Cleveland, OH 44109

Ctr for Women's Health Ab. Access 11710 Shaker Rd. Cleveland, OH 44120

Planned Parenthood 19550 Rockside Rd. Cleveland, OH 44146

Preterm Cleveland – P.P. 12000 Shaker Blvd. Cleveland, OH 44120

Complete Healthcare for Women Dr. Samuel 5888 Cleveland Ave. Columbus, OH 43231

Capital Care Women's Center 4818 Indianola Ave Columbus, OH 43214

Founder's Women's Health Center 1243 E. Broad St. Columbus, OH 43205

Planned Parenthood 3255 E. Main St. Columbus, OH 43213

Women's Medical Center Dr. Martin Haskell, Dr. Neil Strickland, Dr. Roslyn Kade 1401 E. Stroop Rd. Dayton, OH 45429

Ohio Women's Center Fairborn 3162 Presidential Drive Fairborn, OH 45324

Center for Choice II 328 22nd St. Toledo, OH 43604

Toledo Women's Center 1160 W. Sylvania Ave. Toledo, OH 43612

OKLAHOMA – 3 Locations

Abortion Surgery Center Dr. Burns 2453 Wilcox Dr. Norman, OK 73069

Outpatient Services for Women 6112 NW 63rd St. Ok.City, OK 73132

Reproductive Services of Tulsa 6136 E. 32nd PL Tulsa, OK 74135

OREGON – 10 Locations

Planned Parenthood 12220 SW 1st St., # 200 Beaverton, OR 97005

Planned Parenthood 2330 NE Division St., # 7 Bend, OR 97701

The Bours Health Center 539 E 11th Ave Eugene, OR 97401

Dr. Bours Health Center 3303 19th Ave. Forest Grove, OR 97116

Gresham Health Center (PP) 501 NE Hood Ave., Suite 100 Gresham, OR 97030

Bours Health Center Clinics 1520 N.E. Broadway Portland, OR 97232

Downtown Women's Center Inc. 511 SW 10th Ave. # 905 Portland, OR 97205

Lovejoy Surgicenter 933 NW 25th St. Portland, OR 97210

Planned Parenthood – NE Portland Center (Opened 2/14/2010) 3727 NE Martin Luther King Jr. Boulevard Portland, OR 97212

Planned Parenthood – SE Portland Center 3231 SE 50th Ave. Portland, OR 97206

Planned Parenthood 3825 Wolverine Street NE Salem, OR 97305

PENNSYLVANIA – 22 Locations

Allentown Medical Services 2200 W. Hamilton Ave., Ste. 200 Allentown, PA 18104

Allentown Women's Center 1409 Union Blvd., Rear Entrance Allentown, PA 18109

Planned Parenthood 29 North Ninth Street Allentown, PA 18101

Dr. Joel Stein 301 E. City Ave. Ste. 130 Bala Cynwyd, PA 19004

Abortion As An Alternative 5188 Neshaminy Blvd. Bensalem, PA 19020

Hillcrest Women's Medical Center 2709 N. Front Street Harrisburg, PA 17110

Abortion As An Alternative 6043 Germantown Ave. Philadelphia, PA 19144

Gynecological Surgical Consultants 1335 W. Tabor Rd., # 303 Philadelphia, PA 19141

Planned Parenthood 2751 Comly Rd. Philadelphia, PA 19154

Philadelphia Women's Center 777 Appletree St. 7th Floor Philadelphia, PA 19106

Planned Parenthood 1144 Locust St. Philadelphia, PA 19107

Planned Parenthood 2751 Comly Road Philadelphia, PA 19154

Family Women's Medical Society Dr. Kermit Gosnell 3801 Lancaster Ave. Philadelphia, PA 19104

Allegheny Reproductive Health Ctr 200 North Highland FL 2 Pittsburgh, PA 15206

Allegheny Women's Center 121 North Highland Pittsburgh, PA 15206

American Women's Services 320 Fort Duquesne Blvd., Ste. 325 Pittsburgh, PA 15222

Planned Parenthood Women's Hlth. Srvc. 933 Liberty Ave. Pittsburgh, PA 15222

Planned Parenthood 48 S. 4th St. Reading, PA 19602

Reproductive Health Center 1 Medical Center Blvd 4th Fl. Upland, PA 19105

Planned Parenthood 610 Louis Dr. Warminster, PA 18974

P.P. of Chester County 8 S. Wayne St. West Chester, PA 19382

Planned Parenthood 728 S. Beaver St. York, PA 17403

RHODE ISLAND - 2 Locations

Women's Medical Center 1725 Broad St. Cranston, RI 02905

Planned Parenthood 111 Point St. Providence, RI 02903

SOUTH CAROLINA - 3 Locations

Charleston Women's Medical Center 1312 Ashley River Rd. Charleston, SC 29407

Planned Parenthood 2712 Middleburg Dr. # 107 Columbia, SC 29204

Greenville Women's Clinic 1142 Grove Rd. Greenville, SC 29605

SOUTH DAKOTA - 1 Location

Planned Parenthood 6511 W. 41st. St. Sioux Falls, SD 57106

TENNESSEE - 10 Locations

Bristol Obstetrics Gynecology & Family Planning PC aka Bristol Regional Women's Ctr Dr. Adams, Dr. Boyle 2901 West State Street Bristol, TN 37620

Abortion Choice 401 Hudson Dr # 3 Elizabethton , TN 37643

Knoxville Ctr for Reproductive Hlth Dr. Campbell 1547 W. Clinch Ave. Knoxville, TN 37916

Physicians Reproductive Services Dr. Campbell 2011 Laurel Ave. Knoxville, TN 37916

Volunteer Medical Clinic 313 S. Concord St. Knoxville, TN 37916

Memphis Area Med. Ctr for Women 29 S. Bellevue Blvd. Memphis, TN 38104

Memphis Ctr for Reproductive Health 1462 Poplar Ave. Memphis, TN 38104

Planned Parenthood 1407 Union Ave. FL 3 Memphis, TN 38104

P.P. of Mid & East TN 412 Dr. D.B. Todd Jr. Blvd. Nashville, TN 37203

Women's Center 419 Welshwood Dr. Nashville, TN 37222

TEXAS - 41 Locations

Austin Women's Health Center 1902 S. I.H. 35 Austin, TX 78704

International Healthcare Solutions Dr. Kropf 9805 Anderson Mill Rd Austin, TX 78750

Planned Parenthood South Austin 201 East Ben White Blvd. Austin, TX 78704

Whole Women's Health of Austin 8401 N. I.H. 35 Austin, TX 78753

Whole Women's Health 3470 Fannin Suite 3 Beaumont, TX 77701

Planned Parenthood 4112 E. 29th St. Bryan, TX 77802

Dr. Eduardo L Aquino & Dr. Keno 1901 Morgan Ave. Corpus Christi, TX 78404

Abortion Advantage-Dr. Robinson 1929 Record Crossing Rd. Dallas, TX 75235

Northpark Medical Group 8363 Meadow Rd. Dallas, TX 75231

Planned Parenthood 7424 Greenville Ave. # 211 Dallas, TX 75231

Routh St Women's Clinic 4321 N. Central Exp'way Dallas, TX 75235

Southwestern Women's Surgery Center 8616 Greenville Ave. Ste 101 Dallas, TX 75243

Hilltop Women's Reproductive Center Dr. Theard 500 E. Schuster Ave. # B El Paso, TX 79902

Reproductive Services 730 E. Yandell Dr. El Paso, TX 79902

Planned Parenthood 301 S. Henderson St. Fort Worth, TX 76104

Trinity Valley Women's Center Dr. Alan Molson 1717 S. Main St. Fort Worth, TX 76110

West Side Clinic 2011 Las Vegas Trail Fort Worth, TX 76108

Reproductive Services 613 W. Sesame Dr. Harlingen, TX 78550

AAA Concerned Women's Center 7324 Southwest Frwy Houston, TX 77074

A Affordable Women's Medical Center 7007 North Freeway Houston, TX 77076

Aaron Women's Clinic Aka American Women's Clinic 5607 Schumacher Ln Houston, TX 77057

Aaron Women's Surgical Ctr. 2505 North Shepherd Houston, TX 77008

Alto Women's Center 6671 Southwest Freeway STE 450 Houston, TX 77074

Crescent City Women's Center Dr. White 2101 Crawford St. # 312 Houston, TX 77002

Dr. Richard Cunningham 5555 W Loop S. # 200 Houston, TX 77098

Houston Women's Clinic Dr. Bernard Rosenfeld 4820 San Jacinto St. Houston, TX 77004

Planned Parenthood 4600 Gulf Fwy Houston, TX 77023

Planned Parenthood Surgical Srvcs 3601 Fannin St. Houston, TX 77004

Suburban Women's Clinic 3101 Richmond Ave. # 250 Houston, TX 77098

Women's Medical Center Dr. Kaminsky 17070 Red Oak # 505 Houston, TX 77090

Women's Services 4315 Lockwood Dr. # 1 Houston, TX 77026

Killeen Womens Health Center 3106 S. WS Young Dr., Ste. C-302 Killeen, TX 76542

Aaron Women's Health Center 3302 67th St. Lubbock, TX 79413

Whole Women's Health of McAllen 802 S. Main St. McAllen, TX 78501

Planned Parenthood 307 E. Texas Ave. Midland, TX 79701

Alamo Women's Clinic 8600 Wurzbach Rd. # 900E San Antonio, TX 78240

All Women's Medical Center 8600 Wurzbach Rd. # 1206 San Antonio, TX 78240

New Women's Clinic 417 San Pedro Ave. San Antonio, TX 78212

Planned Parenthood 104 Babcock Rd. San Antonio, TX 78201

Private Office Procedures Dr. Dave Kittrell 4499 Medical Dr. # 156 San Antonio, TX 78229

Reproductive Services 5838 Joiner San Antonio, TX 78238

Woman's Choice Quality Health Dr. Dave Kittrell 920 San Pedro Ave. # 100 San Antonio, TX 78212

Planned Parenthood 1927 Columbus Ave. Waco, TX 76701

UTAH – 3 Locations

Mountain View Women's Center 1345 E. 3900 S. # 104 Salt Lake, UT 84124

Utah Women's Clinic 515 S. 400 E. Salt Lake, UT 84111

Wasatch Women's Center 715 E. 3900 S # 203 Salt Lake, UT 84107

VERMONT – 3 Locations

Planned Parenthood 90 Washington St. Barre, VT 05641

Northern New England P.P. 23 Mansfield Ave. Burlington, VT 05401

Planned Parenthood 6 Roberts Ave. Rutland, VT 05701

VIRGINIA – 20 Locations

Alexandria Women's Health Clinic 101 S. Whiting St. # 215 Alexandria, VA 22304

Annandale Women & Family Ctr 2839 Duke St. Alexandria, VA 22314

Charlottesville Medical Ctr for Women 2321 Commonwealth Dr Charlottessville, VA 22901

Charlottesville Obstetrics - P.P. 105 South Pantops Dr. Charlottesville, VA 22911

Planned Parenthood 2964 Hydraulic Road Charlottesville, VA 22901

American Women's Services 8316 Arlington Blvd Fairfax, VA 22031

NOVA Women's Healthcare 10400 Eaton PL. # 515 Fairfax, VA 22030

Falls Church Health Care Center 900 S. Washington St., Ste. 300 Falls Church, VA 22046

Planned Parenthood 370 S. Washington St. # 3 Falls Church, VA 22046

Amethyst Health Center For Women 9380 Forestwood Lane # B Manassas, VA 20110

Penninsula Medical Center for Women 10758 Jefferson Ave. # A Newport News, VA 23601

A Tidewater Womens Health Clinic 891 Norfolk Square Norfolk, VA 23502

Hillcrest Clinic 1600 E. Little Creek Rd. # 235 Norfolk, VA 23518

Norfolk Planned Parenthood 425 W 20th Street # 6 Norfolk, VA 23517

A Capitol Women's Health 1511 Starling Dr. Richmond, VA 23229

Planned Parenthood 201 N Hamilton Street Richmond, VA 23221

Planned Parenthood 2207 Peters Creek Rd. Roanoke, VA 24017

Richmond Med. Ctr. For Women 118 N. Boulevard Richmond, VA 23220

Virginia League for Planned Parenthood 201 N. Hamilton St Richmond, VA 23221

Roanoke Medical Center for Women 1119 2nd St. SW Roanoke, VA 24016

Virginia Women's Wellness 224 Groveland Rd. Virginia Beach, VA 23452

WASHINGTON - 22 Locations

Planned Parenthood- Bellingham Clinic 1530 Ellis St. Bellingham, WA 98225

Planned Parenthood - 1420 156th NE #C Bellvue, WA 98007

Planned Parenthood 623 NE Riddell Road Suite 103 Bremerton, WA 98310

Planned Parenthood 1509 32nd St. Everett, WA 98201

Planned Parenthood 1105 S. 348th St. # B103 Federal Way, WA 98003

Planned Parenthood 6610 NE 181st St. # 2 Kenmore, WA 98028

Planned Parenthood 7426 W. Bonnie PL. Kennewick, WA 99336

Planned Parenthood 402 Legion Way Olympia, WA 98502

Cedar River Clinic 4300 Talbot Rd. S # 403 Renton, WA 98055

All Women's Health North 9730 3rd Ave NE, Suite 200 Seattle, WA 98115

Aurora Medical Services 1001 Broadway, Ste. 320 Seattle, WA 98122

Planned Parenthood 2001 E Madison Seattle, WA 98122

Reproductive Health Specialists Dr. Philip Welch 801 Broadway Ste 628 Seattle, WA 98122

Seattle Medical Clinic Eileen Gibbons 1325 4th Ave. Seattle, WA 98101

Seattle Reproductive Health Anita Johnson Connell, Marci Bowers 1229 Madison Ste 840 Seattle, WA 98104

Planned Parenthood 4500 9th Ave. NE #324 Seattle, WA 98105

PP of Spokane & Whitman Counties 123 E. Indiana Ave. Spokane, WA 99205

All Women's Health Clinic 3711 Pacific Ave. # 200 Tacoma, WA 98418

Cedar River Clinic 1401-A Martin Luther King Way Tacoma, WA 98405

Planned Parenthood 813 Martin Luther King Jr. Way #200 Tacoma, WA 98405

Planned Parenthood 5500 NE 109th Ct., # A Vancouver, WA 98662

Cedar River Clinic 106 East "E" Street Yakima, WA 98901

Planned Parenthood 1117 Tieton Drive Yakima, WA 98902

WEST VIRGINIA – 2 Locations

Kanawha Surgi-Center Dr. Gorli Harish 4803 MacCorkle Ave., SE Charleston, WV 25304

Women's Health Center 510 Washington St. W Charleston, WV 25304

WISCONSIN – 6 Locations

Planned Parenthood 3800 N. Gillette St. Appleton, WI 54913

OB/GYN Assoc. 124 Siegler St. Green Bay, WI 54303

OB/GYN Assoc. 704 S. Webster Green Bay, WI 54301

Planned Parenthood 3706 Orin Road Madison, WI 53704

Affiliated Medical Services 1428 N. Farwell Ave. Milwaukee, WI 53202

Planned Parenthood 302 N. Jackson St. Milwaukee, WI 53202

WYOMING – 1 Location

Emerg-A-Care 982 W. Broadway Jackson, WY 83001

www.ingramcontent.com/pod-product-compliance
Lightning Source LLC
Chambersburg PA
CBHW020243290326
41930CB00038B/234